Gastric Sleeve Cookbook

Easy And Healthy Recipes To Enjoy For All Stages Of Recovery After Weight Loss Surgery

Sara Williams

Limit of Liability

The information in this book is solely for informational purposes, not as a medical instruction to replace the advice of your physician or as a replacement for any treatment prescribed by your physician. The author and publisher do not take responsibility for any possible consequences from any treatment, procedure, exercise, dietary modification, action or application of medication which results from reading or following the information contained in this book.

If you are ill or suspect that you have a medical problem, we strongly encourage you to consult your medical, health, or other competent professional before adopting any of the suggestions in this book or drawing inferences from it.

This book and the author's opinions are solely for informational and educational purposes. The author specifically disclaims all responsibility for any liability, loss, or risk, personal or otherwise which is incurred as a consequence, directly or indirectly, of the use and application of any of the contents of this book.

DEDICATION

To All who desire to live And Eat Healthy

TABLE OF CONTENT

INTRODUCTION

One of the most effective ways to reduce obesity is through Gastric Sleeve Surgery. This is a kind of surgery procedure that is done by reducing the stomach to about 1/10th of the original size. The Gastric Sleeve Surgery is now the most common weight loss surgical operation performed in United States and worldwide.

The surgery is carried out by removing or reducing a portion of the stomach and the remaining is joined together to make it look like a sleeve or banana shape. This surgery helps to limit the size of your stomach to about 1/10th the original size, so that you will eat lesser food and get full quickly.

Differences And Sililarities Between Gastric Bypass And Gastric Sleeve Procedure:

Although, gastric sleeve and gastric bypass are somehow similar in procedures; in both cases the procedures are not reversible, a good reason you need to speak to the doctor about any possible options and side effect. Both surgeries also help to reduce how much food you eat before you get full.

In gastric bypass, the surgeon makes a small pouch that is separated from the rest of the stomach. This is done by cutting one end of the small intestine and attaching a small pouch to allow food bypass the stomach. As a result, the foods you eat will bypass the first section of the small intestine and bottom section of the stomach-, the small intestine will not be able to absolve food you eat, calories intake is reduced which causes you to lose weight.

In gastric Sleeve, the surgery is carried out by removing or reducing a portion of the stomach and the remaining is joined together to make it look like a sleeve or banana shape.

The surgical procedure can be performed in many cases by inserting a medical instrument called lapascope, this instrument has tiny camera attached to it that sends pictures to a monitor, other medical instruments are then inserted through other opening that enable the surgeon operates on the stomach.

Gastric Bypass Diet

A gastric bypass diet is introduced by the doctor or a registered dietitian to patients who has just undergone sleeve gastrectomy or gastric bypass surgery to help them heal and change from their former eating pattern. Your dietitian or doctor will need to give a broad explanation on your diet changes, what type of food to eat and meal portion that is safe for you.

Why gastric Bypass diet:

Gastric bypass diet plays an important role in safely recovering after undergoing gastric bypass surgery.

It can help you to avoid gaining weight.

Helps to avoid any side effects or complications as a result of the surgery

Helps you adapt to new eating habit of smaller meal portion that is easy for your stomach to digest

Help your stomach heal quickly without overstretching by food

Preparing Before The Surgery

Before you qualify for gastric sleeve surgery, you will need to meet with a bariatric surgeon and their registered nutritionist; they will explain in details to you all you need to know about the surgery. Your bariatric surgeon also needs to consider many factors before you can be allowed to have the surgery; like, your overall health, overall body mass index (BMI). Patients are usually advised by surgeon to complete Weight management program before gastric sleeve surgery. While the expected body mass index (BMI) is at least 40, people that are too heavy may not be qualified for gastric surgery to avoid any complications associated with postoperative. Other medical complications that could be a result of weight gain, such as liver disease, diabetes, heart disease etc.

Before the bariatric surgery, surgeon's needs to be sure the patient can be committed to a new eating habit over a long period of time. They will also provide you with a clear diet plan for each stage of the diet. The diet is aimed at helping you recover safely without getting over-stretched by food and also build a new basis for healthy eating habits. However, there's no specific period of time following a diet plan for gastric sleeve post-operation, but experts have confirmed it is more effective to stay on a low carb diet than low fat diet in the short term (2–6 weeks), focusing more on people with metabolic syndrome or nonalcoholic fatty liver disease.

Getting ready for gastric sleeve surgery takes months of preparation, you will have to work closely with a team of medical professionals to assist you build the skills required for a successful operation. Some of the skills will require the service of psychologists, doctors and surgeons, dietitians, and exercise specialists.

Psychologists: Most times our emotions can easily play a hard trick on us without being able to control it. A Psychologist should be readily available to help you deal with the emotional part. People differs in many ways, it might not be so difficult for some patient to quickly feel better after a weight loss surgery, others might not find it as easy as others or probably find themselves struggling due to anxiety or depression as a result of the surgery. Psychologists are readily available to help envisage coping strategies to deal with any emotions, stress or worries as a result of the surgery.

Doctors and surgeons: You will also need to meet with team of surgeons and doctors several months before the surgery. Their duty is to examine and explain in details what to expect post and pre surgery, any possible side effect or complications that can likely occur after the surgery.

Dietitians: Your diet plays a very important role on how quickly you recover after the surgery. Dietitians will provide you with a clear diet plan for each stage of the diet, how to embrace new healthy eating habits; like healthy portion sizes and good nutrition. They may also need to talk to you or any family member you may rely on for food because the size of the stomach will be permanently decreases after gastric sleeve surgery. Dietitians will need to fully explain what to eat and not to, how to gradually make changes to your eating pattern for the rest of your life.

Exercise specialists:
These experts help you to develop a workout routine that will not over stress you, helping you become more active before and after the surgery. Exercising before surgery month helps patients' recovery faster and be in a good spirit for the operation. It also makes it easy for patients to return to working out after surgery. All you need is to go steadily; a gradual process will not let you overstress yourself back into your exercise routine.

You have to understand that this surgery will forever change the way you eat. For a successful operation it is important not only for a person to change what they eat but also need to make few adjustments on how they eat it. Dietitians will brief and instruct you about what types of food to eat or not to, how to gradually make changes with portion size for each meal.

It is mandatory to follow this new diet stage by stage before you get a green light on eating solid foods again. How long it takes to move from one stage to the other depends on the patient body ability to heal and adjust quickly to the new eating pattern. In most case you should be able to eat solid food after three months of surgery.

WHAT TO EAT AFTER THE SURGERY

Clear Liquid:

After the first day of the surgery you are expected to drink clear liquid, and once you are able to handle that, you then proceed to drinking other liquid for the next seven days, such as:

Sugar-free

Milk (skim or 1 percent)

Decaffeinated tea or coffee

Unsweetened juice

Noncarbonated clear liquids

Broth

Sugar-free popsicles or gelatin

Pureed Food: Once you get a green light after you are able to handle clear liquid well, you can start drinking protein shakes and pureed foods (mashed up) for the next four weeks. The puree should be in form of thick liquid or smooth paste, free of any solid pieces.

You can eat up to 3 to 6 meals a day consisting of about 4 to 6 tablespoons of puree food per servings. Take your time and eat slowly, about half an hour per meal.

Your puree food should consist of any foods that will puree well, such as:
Skim milk with protein powder
Strained cream soups
Protein supplements
Cooked vegetables and soft fruits
Cooked cereal
Pureed pineapples, apricots, peaches, peaches, melons
Mashed nonfat or Low fat cottage cheese
Soft scrambled eggs
Cottage cheese
Mashed bananas
Pureed Poultry, lean ground meat, or fish

Solid foods that are well blended with a liquid, such as:
Broth
Water
No sugar added juice
Skim milk

Soft Food: Patients can start introducing soft food after the first month of surgery or once your doctor says it's okay. You can eat up to 3 to 5 meals a day consisting of about 1/3 to 1/2 cup of soft food per servings.

Soft food should consist of:
Cooked vegetables, without skin

Rice
Cooked or dried cereal
Sliced or grated Cottage cheese
Cooked or canned vegetables
Poached or hard boiled eggs
Skinless fresh fruit –apples, peaches, pears
Cereals moistened in unsweetened skim milk
Flaked fish
Ground lean meat or poultry
White rice, boiled pasta or noodles
Fresh and ripe bananas

Solid Food: Once you get a green light after 2 or 3 months of eating soft food, you can gradually move on to eating solid foods.
You can eat up to 3 meals a day consisting of about 1 to 1-1/2 cups per servings. Take your time and eat slowly, it is advised to stop eating even before you are completely full- about 30 minutes per meal.

It's not a bad idea to introduce new food, but go slowly, one at a time. Some foods may cause you pain, puke or vomit. Tolerance depends on individual's body system. Have a regular discussion with your dietitian about your choice of food and how your body reacts to it.

Here are some of the foods that can cause problems at this stage:
Red meat
Nuts and seeds
Carbonated drinks
Highly spicy or seasoned foods
Fried foods
Popcorn
Tough meats or meats with gristle
Cooked fibrous vegetables, such as broccoli, celery, cabbage or corn

Raw vegetables

Breads

You might be able to tolerate some of these foods over time based on your doctor's guidance.

At All Stages after The Surgery You Most:

Keeping in mind that food needs to be chewed very slowly and thoroughly before you swallow to avoid dumping syndrome.
Dumping syndrome occur when food are not properly chewed before swallowing or occur as a result of large particles of food entering the small intestine too rapidly which can cause:
Dizziness
Nausea
Vomiting
Diarrhea
Abdominal pain
Sweating

Take your time and eat slowly, about 30 minutes per meal.
Do not drink liquid within meals, only 30 minutes after or before food
All patients take multi-vitamin and mineral supplements daily according to your physician directions. Your body may not able to absorb all the required nutrients from the food you eat.
Do not take high-calorie sodas and snack
Eat lean, protein-rich foods daily even before other foods in your meal.
Avoid foods that are high in sugar and fat.
Limit caffeine, which can cause dehydration
Avoid alcohol

Gastric sleeve surgery can be associated with any of these complications, especially if you do not follow the diet properly; eat food you are not supposed to eat or eat too much. This includes:

Dumping syndrome:
Dumping syndrome is one of the most common symptoms of gastric sleeve surgery. This can occur when food are not properly chewed before swallowing or as a result of large particles of food entering the small intestine too rapidly. Dumping syndrome can cause dizziness, nausea, vomiting, diarrhea, abdominal pain, sweating.

Dehydration:
If you do not drink enough water through the day, you can become dehydrated; you are expected to drink about 1.9 liters (64 ounces) of water and other fluids a day.

Constipation: You need enough physical activity to avoid constipation, more so, your food should not be fiber or fluid deficient.

Blocked opening of your stomach pouch: Even after you have followed the diet precisely, chances are food can still accumulate at the opening of your stomach pouch. When you feel pain in your abdomen, experience nausea or vomiting, these can be common signs that there is a blockage in the opening of your stomach pouch. Call your doctor if these symptoms last for more than two days.
Failure to lose weight or weight gain: If you fail to lose weight or continue to gain more weight, talk to your dietitian or doctor.

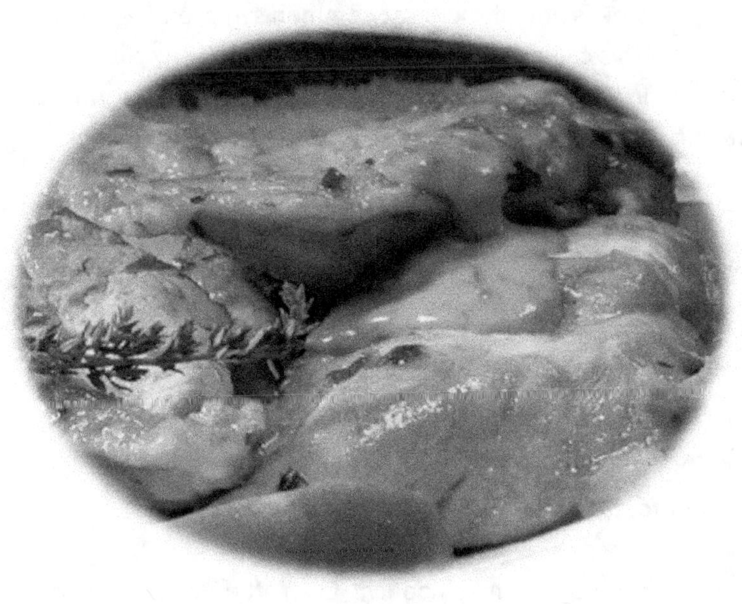

Great Protein Shake

Prep time: 5 minutes

Ready time: 5 minutes

Servings: 2

INGREDIENTS

1 tsp of Rum extract

1/4 tsp of Nutmeg

1/4 tsp of Cinnamon

2 cup of ice

2 Premier Protein Shake Vanilla

INSTRUCTIONS

1. Place the protein Vanilla and ice cubes into a bender.

2. Add in the cinnamon plus rum extract. Blend until mixture is smooth.

Top with a sprinkle of nutmeg and serve. Enjoy!

Nutrition per servings

Calories: 162kcal; Carbohydrates: 4g; Protein: 30g; Fat: 3g

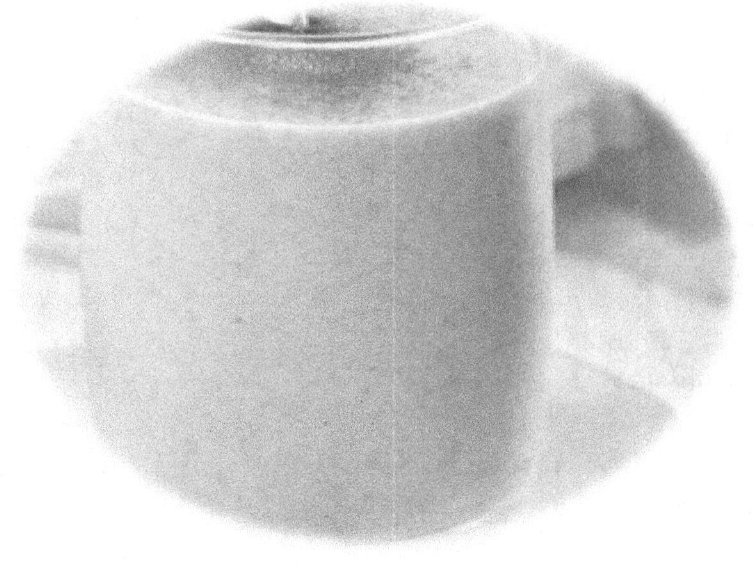

Prep time: 5 minutes

Ready time: 5 minutes

Servings: 1

INGREDIENTS

1/2 tsp of lime juice

1/4 cup of coconut milk

1/2 cups of fresh or frozen blueberries

1 fresh mint leaves

1/4 cup of grapefruit

INSTRUCTIONS

1. Combine together the blueberries, lime juice, coconut milk and grapefruit in a high-power blender.

2. Pour into serving glass and garnish with the mint leaves.

Nutrition per servings

Calories: 247kcal; Protein: 30g; Fat: 2.23g

Fancy Smoothie

Prep time: 5 minutes

Ready time: minutes

Servings: 2

INGREDIENTS

2/3 cup of fresh orange juice

¼ ripe avocado, peeled and chopped

5 tbsp of low-fat coconut milk

Small handful (10 g) of spinach leaves

1 dessert pear

1 apple, core and cut into small chunks

INSTRUCTIONS

1. Place the apple, orange juice, coconut milk, avocado and spinach in a smoothie maker or blender. Pulse until mixture is smooth. Serve in glass and enjoy!

Nutrition per servings
Calories: 321kcal; Carbohydrates: 12g; Protein: 5g; Fat: 12g

Mayo Mango Protein Shake

Ready time: 5 minutes
Servings: 2
INGREDIENTS
1/2 packet of True Orange flavoring
1/2 tbsp of banana flavored syrup (sugar-free)
A squirt of lemon juice
Ice cubes
1/2 Premier Protein 5.5 oz. Vanilla Shake
1-1 1/2 peach segments (frozen)
1/4 cup of fresh cut mango, cubed
1/2 cup of unflavored Greek yogurt
INSTRUCTIONS
1. Combine the entire ingredients apart from the ice in a powerful blender, blend for 1-2 minutes. Add ice and blend for 1 minute extra until smooth.

Greek Peach Drink

Prep time: 5 minutes

Ready time: 5 minutes

Servings: 2

INGREDIENTS

1 cup of frozen Peaches

2 cup ice

1 cup of frozen Mango

1 cup of Skim Milk

2 cup of nonfat Greek Style Yogurt

INSTRUCTIONS

1. Add the frozen fruit and yogurt in a blender. Add in the Skim milk and ice. Mix until smooth and enjoy.

Nutrition per servings

Calories: 288kcal; Carbohydrates: 22g; Protein: 30g; Fat: 1.56g

Oat Protein Drink

Prep time: 5 minutes

Ready time: 5 minutes

Servings: 3

INGREDIENTS

1/2 Tbsp of chia seeds

3/4 - 1 cups of unsweetened almond milk

1/2 - 1 Tbsp of cacao powder (to taste)

 (Optional) 1/2 - 1 pitted dates or maple syrup

1/2 frozen ripe banana

1/8 cup gluten-free oats

1 Tbsp of hemp seeds

1 Tbsp of natural salted peanut, almond or cashew butter

INSTRUCTIONS

1. Add the frozen banana, oats, hemp seeds, nut butter of choice, almond milk, chia seeds and cacao powder in a high-powered blender and blend on high speed until smooth and creamy, scraping down the sides.

Taste to adjust flavor if needed. Add maple syrup or dates for sweetness, cacao powder for color, almond milk to thin and butter for saltiness or creaminess or. Best serve and enjoy immediately. Keep in the refrigerator covered up to 1 day.

Nutrition per servings
Calories: 307kcal; Carbohydrates: 21g; Protein: 10g;

Berries Parfait

Prep time: 5 minutes
Ready time: 5 minutes
Servings: 2
INGREDIENTS
2 medium strawberries, removed top and chop
4 tbsp of blueberries
1 cup of light vanilla yogurt or nonfat Greek yogurt
4 tbsp of raspberries
2 or 4 packets of sugar substitute, or to taste
1/2 tsp of vanilla extract
INSTRUCTIONS
1. Mix together the raspberries, sugar substitute, blueberries and vanilla in a bowl.
2. Add ¼ of the light vanilla yogurt into an 8-oz glass. Pour in 1/2 the mixture on top the yogurt. Add the remaining berries and yogurt.

Nutrition per servings:
Calories: 110kcal; Carbohydrates: 18g; Protein: 4g; Fat: 3g

Prep time: 5 minutes

Ready time: 5 minutes

Servings: 2

INGREDIENTS

2 packet of no-calorie sweetener

8-9 oz. unsweetened vanilla almond milk

2 scoop of Syntrax Nectar Caribbean Cooler protein

16 ice cubes

(Optional) Sugar-free caramel sauce, fat-free whipped cream

1 sliced of banana (frozen)

INSTRUCTIONS

1. Combine the entire ingredients together in a powerful blender apart from the ice, blend for 1-2 minutes. Add ice and blend for 1 minute extra until smooth.

Nutrition per servings:

Calories: 311kcal; Carbohydrates: 17g; Protein: 22g; Fat: 7g

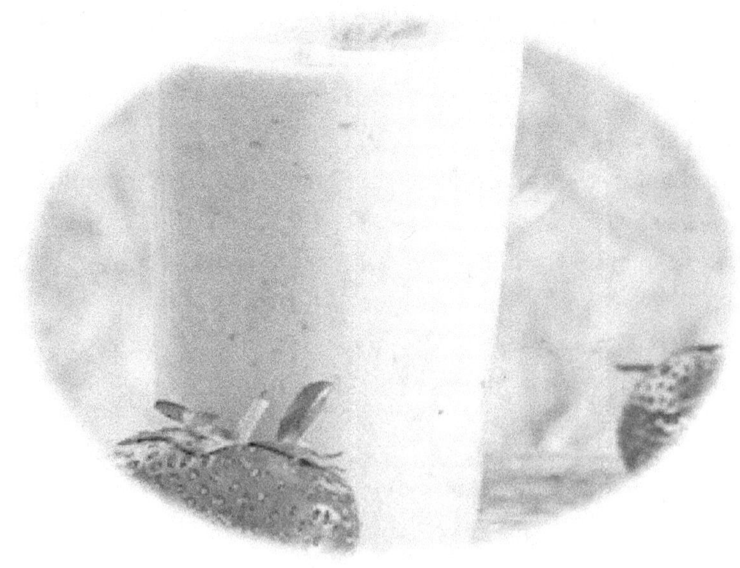

Super Splendid Soup

Prep time: 5 minutes

Cook time: 12 minutes

Servings: 2

INGREDIENTS

1 tbsp of shiro miso paste

Nori seaweed to serve

1 tbsp of Nutra Organics Collagen Powder

1 tbsp of wheat free tamari soy sauce

1 sliced spring onions to serve

2 cups of filtered water

1 1/2 garlic cloves, smashed

Small 5g ginger knob, finely sliced

INSTRUCTIONS

1. Bring water to the boil over medium high heat in a large stainless steel pot.

2. Add in the smashed garlic and sliced ginger, reduce heat and let it simmer for about 10 minutes. Turn heat off.

3. Add in the miso paste, tamari and Collagen Powder, stir everything to mix well.

Taste and adjust the garlic and ginger if needed. Fold in the onions just before you serve.

4. Serve soup in bowls and garnish with nori seaweed.

Nutrition per servings:

Calories: 32kcal; Carbohydrates: 2.1g Protein: 3g; Fat: 0.55

Creamy Fruity Smoothie

Prep time: 5 minutes

Ready time: 5 minutes

Servings: 4

INGREDIENTS

2 dash of black pepper

2 dash of ground clove and cardamom (optional plus spice)

2 dash of ground nutmeg

1/2 cup of fresh carrot juice (optional)

2 dash of ground cinnamon

2 cup of frozen ripe banana (sliced)

2 Tbsp of fresh ginger (plus more to taste)

1 tsp of ground turmeric powder

2 cup of light coconut or almond milk (Best use full-fat coconut)

INSTRUCTIONS

1. Add the coconut milk, banana, cinnamon, black pepper, nutmeg, ginger and turmeric to a high-powered blender and blend on high speed until you have smooth and creamy mixture.

2. Add fresh carrot juice, cardamom and clove (if using). Add more frozen banana if too thin and more water or coconut milk if too thick.

2. Taste and adjust flavor as desired. Serve and enjoy!

Nutrition per servings:
Calories: 274kcal; Carbohydrates: 22g; Protein: 15g; Fat: 11g

Pumpkin Creamy Shake

Prep time: 5 minutes

Ready time: 5 minutes

Servings: 2

INGREDIENTS:

Whipped cream and a sugar-free caramel drizzle (Optional)

Ice

4 tablespoon of sugar-free English Toffee syrup

1/2 teaspoon of sugar-free pumpkin pie or pumpkin pie spice

2 ounces of canned pumpkin puree (not the pie filling)

2 scoop of vanilla protein powder

2 cup of nonfat milk

INSTRUCTIONS

1. Combine the entire ingredients apart from the ice in a powerful blender, blend for 1-2 minutes. Add ice and blend for 1 minute extra until smooth.

Nutrition per servings:
Calories: 408kcal; Protein: 40.4g; Fat: 9.39g

Prep time: 5 minutes

Ready time: 5 minutes

Servings: 3

INGREDIENTS

2 fresh pitted dates or 1/2 tbsp of raw honey

1/2 tsp of vanilla extract

1 tbsp of Coconut butter or tahini

1/4 tsp of sea salt

1/2 cup of pumpkin seeds (soaked)

3 cups of filtered water

1/2 tsp of organic matcha green tea powder

INSTRUCTIONS

 1. Combine the dates, pumpkin seeds, matcha, coconut butter, vanilla, water and salt in a high-powered blender and blend for 30 seconds to 1 minute until smooth and creamy.

2. Strain through a fine sieve and transfer Into a glass jug. Refrigerate until needed.

Nutrition per servings:

Calories: 278kcal; Carbohydrates: 11g Protein: 7g; Fat: 10g

PUREE FOOD STAGE

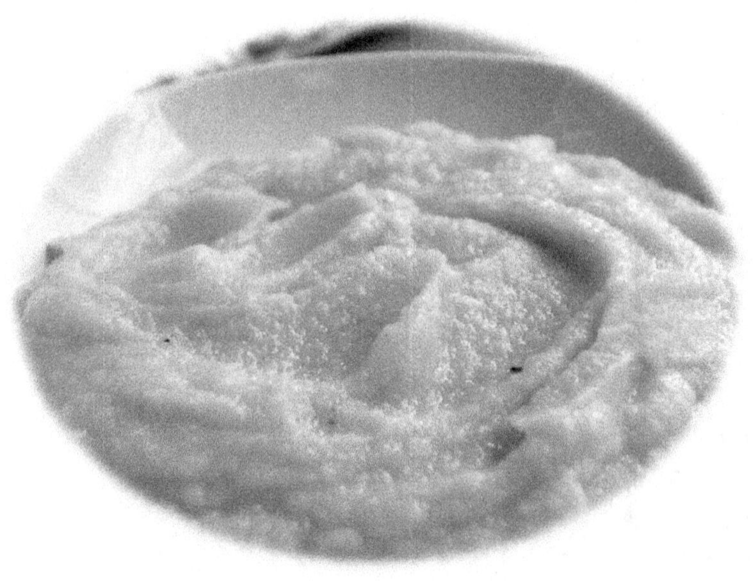

Purred Egg

Prep time: 5 minutes

Ready time: 5 minutes

Servings: 1

INGREDIENTS

Salt and pepper to taste

1 hard-boiled eggs, sliced

1/2 tbsp of plain Greek-style yogurt

1/2 tbsp of reduced-fat mayonnaise

INSTRUCTIONS

1. Chop the egg into small pieces in a food processor.

2. Add in the Greek yogurt, mayonnaise, and seasonings and blend well until smooth.

Nutrition per servings

Calories: 176kcal; Carbohydrates: 4.6g; Protein: 9.3g; Fat: 13.2g

Pureed Chicken With Cheese

Prep time: 5 minutes

Ready time: 5 minutes

Servings: 2

INGREDIENTS

3 tbsp of tomato sauce

1/4 tsp of pepper

1/4 tsp of salt

1/2 cup of canned chicken

2 tsp of Italian seasoning

Optional: ricotta cheese or low-fat cottage cheese

INSTRUCTIONS

1. Place the canned chicken, pepper, tomato sauce, Italian seasoning and salt in a small blender or blend using the back of a fork until ingredients are finely blended and smooth. Add in the cheese if using.

2. Transfer into bowl and place in the microwave for about 30 seconds.

Nutrition per servings
Carbohydrates: 3g; Protein: 13g; Fat: 4g

Smooth Lemon Salmon

Prep time: 5 minutes
Ready time: 5 minutes
Servings: 2

INGREDIENTS

1 tsp of dried dill
1/4 tsp of salt
2 tbsp of fresh lemon juice
1/4 tsp of pepper
4 tbsp of 0% fat, plain Greek yogurt
5 ounces of fresh smoked salmon

INSTRUCTIONS

1. Place the smoked salmon, dried dill, lemon juice, salt and pepper into a food processor. Blend until the fish is finely diced. Stir in Greek Yogurt until smooth.

Nutrition per servings
Calories: kcal; Carbohydrates: 2g; Protein: 13g; Fat: 3g

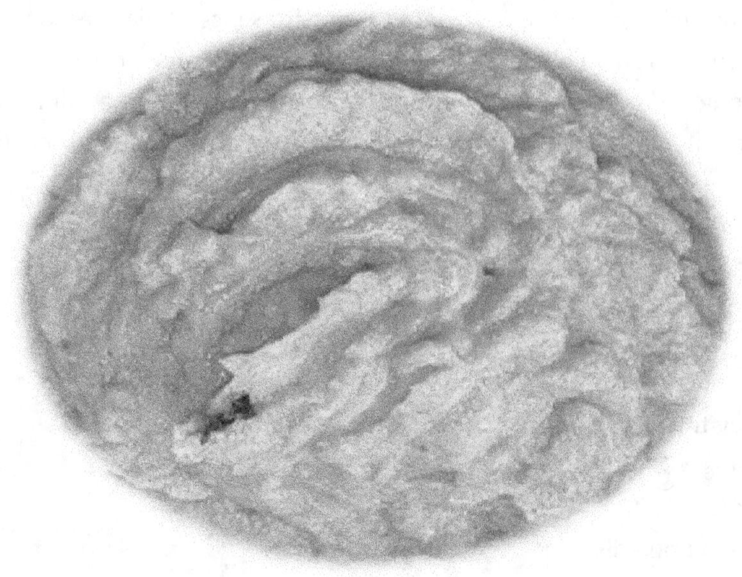

Garlic Soft Salmon Puree

Prep time: 10 minutes

Ready time: 5 minutes

Servings: 2

INGREDIENTS

1 tbsp of reduced-fat mayonnaise

1/16 tsp of garlic powder

1/2 tsp of lemon juice

2.5 oz canned salmon, drained (or cooked salmon or tuna fillet)

INSTRUCTIONS

1. Drop the salmon into a food processor.

2. Add in lemon juice, mayonnaise and garlic and process until mixture is smooth. Taste and adjust lemon and garlic to your desired taste.

Nutrition per servings

Calories: 88kcal; Carbohydrates: 1g; Protein: 11g; Fat: 4g

Tuna Relish Salad Puree

Prep time: 5 minutes

Ready time: 5 minutes

Servings: 2

INGREDIENTS

1/2-1 tbsp of low-fat mayonnaise

1 tbsp of plain Greek Yogurt

1 tsp of relish

Salt and pepper to taste

8 oz. can of tuna packed in water

INSTRUCTIONS

1. Add the relish and tuna chunks in a small food processor and process into small pieces.

2. Pour the relish/tuna mixture into a mixing bowl. Add in the yogurt and mayonnaise, stir to combine; Season with salt and pepper.

Nutrition per servings: Serve in 1/4 cup (2 oz)

Calories: 78kcal; Carbohydrates: 1.7g; Protein: 10.5g; Fat: 2.9g

Butternut Maple Puree

Prep time: 10 minutes
Ready time: 15 minutes
Servings: 4
INGREDIENTS
Cayenne pepper
1/2 tbs of maple syrup
1/2 tbs of butter
1/2-1 tbs of water
1/2 Butternut squash, peeled and remove seed (cut in 1 inch cubes)
INSTRUCTIONS
1. Add the squash cubes in a microwave-safe bowl, cover with paper towel.
2. Place bowl in the microwave for 5 minutes, remove and stir. Cover again with paper towel and place back in the microwave, cook further for 5 minutes or until soft; Drain.
3. Blend together the squash, water, maple syrup, butter and cayenne pepper in blender until smooth.

Nutrition per servings: Serve in 1/4 cup (2 oz)
Calories: 78kcal; Carbohydrates: 5g; Protein: 5g

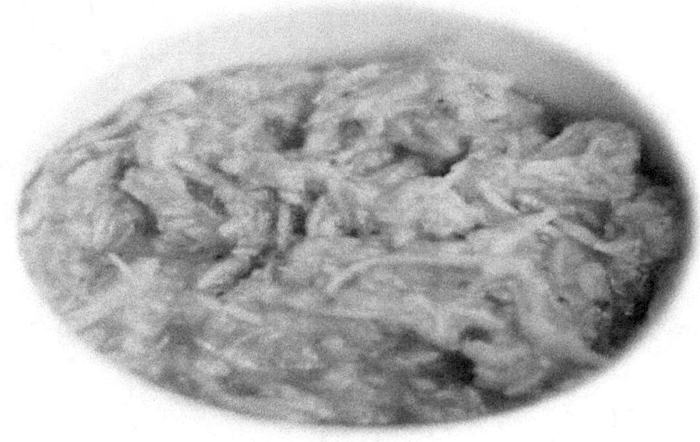

Prep time: 10 minutes

Ready time: 20 minutes

Servings: 2

INGREDIENTS

1/8 tsp of salt

1/4 cup of nonfat milk

1/2 large Russet potato, cubed

1/4 cup of shredded low fat cheddar cheese

1 cups of vegetable or chicken stock

1/2 large shallot, minced

1/2 large head broccoli or 1/2 pound fresh (frozen can do the job also)

1/2 tbsp of butter

INSTRUCTIONS

1. Start by chopping the broccoli into 1- inch pieces and set aside.

2. Combine the butter and minced shallot in a pot and place over medium heat. Stir together until smooth and softened.

3. Add the vegetable or chicken stock, potato, broccoli and salt to the pot. Simmer for about 15 minutes or until tender. Remove from heat and add the milk.

4. Blend mixture using a hand held blender until it's smooth. Stir in the cheese using a wooden spatula until melted.

Nutrition per servings:

Calories: 150kcal; Carbohydrates: 16g; Protein: 10 g; Fat: 5g

Prep time: 5 minutes

Ready time: 5 minutes

Servings: 2

INGREDIENTS

4 tbsp of chicken or vegetable broth

2 eggs

2 tbsp of unflavored whey protein powder

Salt and pepper to taste

6 tbsp of green enchilada sauce, divided

1 cup of black beans, rinsed

INSTRUCTIONS

Black Bean Puree

1. Add the black beans and enchilada sauce in a saucepan and cook over medium heat; stirring for 2 minutes. Once heated through, pour in the broth.

2. Blend the black bean mixture in the blender or use a hand held blender and blend until mixture is smooth. Transfer to a bowl and allow cooling slightly. Stir in the protein powder until well mixed. Cover with a foil and keep warm. Keep leftover in the refrigerator another meal.

Scrambled Egg

3. Place a non-stick pan over medium heat. Whisk the egg in a mixing bowl until frothy.

4. Pour half the beaten egg into hot pan. Sprinkle top with pepper and salt. Gently stir egg around using a rubber spatula and cook until everything is almost cooked but still a bit running. Fold the egg over itself and transfer onto a plate. Repeat steps with the second half.

5. Add 1 tablespoon the puree on top each egg and serve.

Nutrition per servings:

Carbohydrates: 6g; Protein: 11g; Fat: 5g

Prep time: 5 minutes

Servings: 4

INGREDIENTS

1/4 tsp of nutmeg

2 tsp of vanilla extract

Sugar substitute to taste

1/2 tsp of cinnamon

2 cup of light vanilla yogurt or plain nonfat yogurt

1/4 tsp of ground ginger

1 tsp of liquid butter extract

1/4 tsp of allspice

1 cup of canned pumpkin

INSTRUCTIONS

1. Combine together the ingredients in a mixing bowl. Chill in the refrigerator until ready to serve

Nutrition per servings:

Calories: 90kcal; Carbohydrates: 13g; Protein: 5g; Fat: 2g

Beans Salsa Pureed

Prep time: 5 minutes

Cook time: 5 minutes

Servings: 4

INGREDIENTS

1 scoop of unflavored whey protein powder

2 tbsp of chicken broth

2 tbsp of salsa of choice

1 (15 ounces) can of pinto beans

INSTRUCTIONS

1. In a small sauce pan, mix together the entire ingredients over medium high heat. Stir periodically for few minutes until warmed.

2. Pour everything to a blender and blend for a few minutes on high until smooth. Serve! Store any leftovers a storage containers.

Nutrition per servings:

Calories. kcal, Carbohydrates. 15g, Protein. 11g, Fat. 1g

Smoked Salmon

Prep time: 5 minutes

Cook time: 5 minutes

Servings: 1

INGREDIENTS

1/8 tsp of pepper

1/8 tsp of salt

1 tbsp of fresh lemon juice

1/2 tsp of dried dill

2 tbsp of 0% fat, plain Greek yogurt

2.5 ounces of fresh smoked salmon

INSTRUCTIONS

1. Add all the ingredients into a blender or food processor except Greek Yogurt and blend until fish is nicely diced.
2. Stir in the Greek Yogurt using a spoon until smooth.

Nutrition per servings:
Calories: kcal; Carbohydrates: 2g; Protein: 13g; Fat: 3g

Healthy Popsicles

Prep time: 5 minutes
Ready time: 7 minutes
Servings: 4
INGREDIENTS
1/4 tsp of ground ginger
1 tbsp of black chia seeds
1/8 cup of water
1 ripe, yellow large cling peaches peeled and seed removed
1 scoops BiPro USA Unflavored protein powder
1/4 cup of no-calorie sweetener of choice
INSTRUCTIONS
1. Whisk the peaches, protein powder, ginger, water and sweetener together in a high power blender and blend until smooth.
2. Taste and check if the ginger taste is strong enough, if not, add more pinch of the ginger. If too strong, add more peaches.
3. Now, check if it's sweet enough (It should be slightly over-sweet before freezing because freezing naturally reduces the sweetness)
4. Transfer mixture into a bowl and place the chia seeds. Stir well, cover and refrigerate for 2 hours.
5. Stir once again then fill the Popsicle mold with the mixture. Freeze for two hours.
6. Remove Popsicle mold by running the mold under lukewarm water until easy to remove.

Nutrition per servings:
Calories: 78kcal; Carbohydrates: 5g; Protein: 7.2g; Fat: 1.8g

Mocha Pudding

Prep time: 10 minutes

Ready time: 60 minutes

Servings: 2

INGREDIENTS

1/2 tbsp of unsweetened cocoa powder

2 tbsp of whipped cream

1/16 tsp of peppermint extract

1 cup of milk

(Optional) 1-1 1/2 sugar-free peppermints

1/2 (0.25 oz.) box of instant chocolate pudding mix (sugar-free)

1/2 tsp of Cafe Bustelo instant decaffeinated espresso

1 servings of Chocolate protein powder, BiPro USA

INSTRUCTIONS

1. In a mixing bowl, whisk together the protein powder, pudding mix, cocoa powder and instant espresso until well combined.

2. Add in the peppermint extract and milk, then beat with a hand mixer on medium speed for a few seconds, then increase speed until smooth. Scrapping the sides of the bowl as needed to mix all ingredients.

3. Taste, and if the mint is not strong as desired, add just a little drop of extract. (Do not over use)

4. Divide the mixture evenly between two cups. Chill in the refrigerator for one hour.

5. Serve, topped with crushed sugar-free peppermint pieces and whipped cream, if desired. Serve with sugar-free crushed peppermint pieces and whipped cream, if desired.

Nutrition per servings:
Calories: 192kcal; Carbohydrates: 12g; Protein: 12g; Fat: 8g

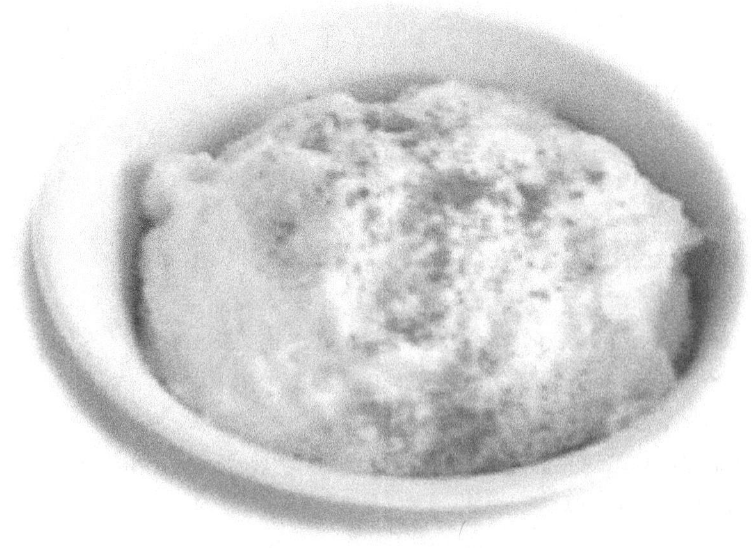

Quick Cheesecake

Ready in: 5 minutes

Servings: 1/4 cup

INGREDIENTS

1 package sugar-free cheesecake pudding mix

1 cup of plain fat-free Greek yogurt

INSTRUCTIONS

1. Combine both ingredients in a high speed blender and puree until mixture is smooth.

Nutrition per servings:

Protein: 7 grams

Avocado Beans Jalapeño Spread

Prep time: 5 minutes

Servings: 6

INGREDIENTS

¼ tsp of salt

½ tsp of green Tabasco sauce

½ green jalapeño, seeded and chopped

1 ½ tbsp of fresh lime juice

2 large sprigs of cilantro

2/3 cup of cannellini or white beans, rinsed and drained

1 ripe, medium-sized avocado

INSTRUCTIONS

1. Blend the entire ingredients in food processor or blender until smooth and creamy.

Use as topping or dip for vegetables or chicken.

Nutrition per servings:

Calories: 85kcal; Carbohydrates: 4g; Protein: 2g; Fat: 5g

Creamy Cauliflower Bowl

Prep time: 5 minutes

Ready time: 8 minutes

Servings: 2

INGREDIENTS

2 tsp of extra-virgin olive oil

1/4 tsp of garlic salt

1/2 tsp of butter, salted

1/2 (about 3-3 1/2") large head of cauliflower (Break into small pieces)

1/4 tsp of black pepper

1/6 cup of low-fat buttermilk

6 garlic cloves (cooked/steamed with cauliflower)
INSTRUCTIONS
1. Toss the cauliflower along with the garlic into a heat-proof bowl, add
1/6 cup of water and cover; microwave cauliflower until very tender,
about 5 minutes or so.
2. Transfer the cooked cauliflower into a food processor. Crush the
garlic cloves with a garlic press and place in the food processor.
3. Add 1 teaspoons olive oil, buttermilk, butter, pepper and garlic salt
into the food processor and process until smooth and creamy. Drizzle
with top with remaining olive oil and serve.

Nutrition per servings
Calories: 113kcal; Carbohydrates: 11g; Protein: 5g; Fat: 6g

Light Chicken Salad`
Prep time: 5 minutes
Ready time: 5 minutes
Servings: 1/2 cup
INGREDIENTS
4 tbsp of Light Mayonnaise
Pinch of black pepper
1/4 tsp of onion powder
2 cooked chicken breast
1/4 tsp of celery salt
4 tbsp of plain Greek style yogurt
INSTRUCTIONS
1. Grind the chicken breast in a food processor until consistency is fine.
Stir in mayonnaise, yogurt, onion powder, celery, pepper and salt until
smooth.

Nutrition per servings:
Calories: 84kcal; Carbohydrates: 0.9g; Protein: 10.7g; Fat: 4g

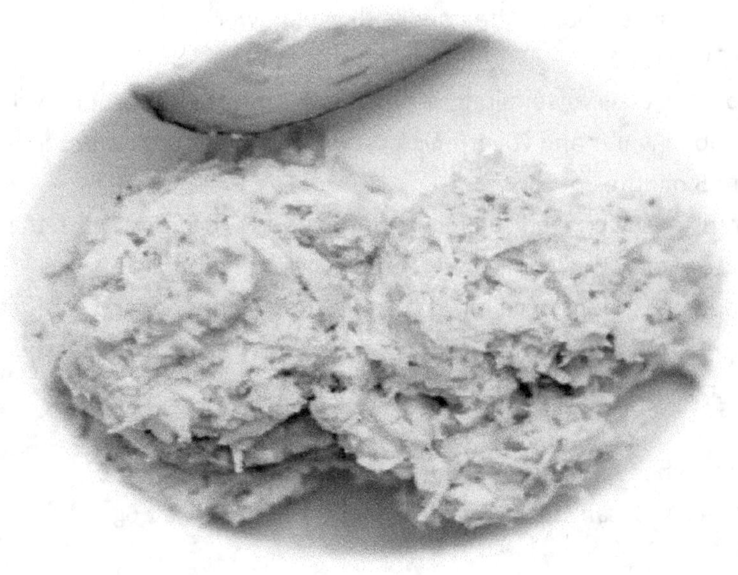

Grilled Onion Eggplant

Prep time: 5 minutes

Ready time: 50 minutes

Servings: 4

INGREDIENTS

2 tbsp of lemon juice

4 tsp of olive oil

4 tbsp of chopped fresh flat-leaf parsley

250 grams eggplant

1 finely chopped medium onion

Salt and pepper to taste

4 tsp of crushed garlic

INSTRUCTIONS

1. Heat-up the oven to 350 degrees F.

2. Add the eggplant in a baking pan and bake in the oven for 45 minutes or until soft. Set aside to cool slightly before pilling the skin.

3. Chop eggplants roughly and add into a food processor along with the remaining ingredients, blend until creamy and smooth; served hot or cold.

Nutrition per servings:
Calories: 131kcal; Carbohydrates: 15g; Protein: 3.7g; Fat: 4g

Broccoli And Sweet Potato Puree

Prep time: 5 minutes

Ready time: 15 minutes

Servings: 4

INGREDIENTS

1/4 tsp of ground coriander

1/4 tbsp of grated orange rind

1 tbsp of chopped fresh flat-leaf parsley

1 tbsp of white wine vinegar

250 grams sweet potatoes, peeled and chopped

1/4 tsp of ground cumin

1/2 tsp of honey

100 grams of broccoli, cut in to florets

1/2 cup of water

INSTRUCTIONS

1. Pour water into a pot, add the sweet potato and bring to a boil. Reduce heat and let it simmer for about 10 minutes.

2. Add in the broccoli florets and cook until very tender, about 5 minutes. Remove pot from heat.

3. Puree the cooked broccoli along with the cooking liquid and spices in a blender or food processor until smooth. Do this in batches.

Nutrition per servings:
Calories: 67kcal; Carbohydrates: 11g; Protein: 3.7g; Fat: 2.23g

Prep time: 10 minutes

Ready time: 1 hour 40 minutes

Servings: 4 ounce per servings

INGREDIENTS

2 ounces (2 cubes) of minced onions

1/2 tsp of salt

Taco seasoning packet

6 oz. cups of cooked chicken [chicken in water can]

1/2 tsp of garlic powder

1/2 cup of red kidney beans

1/4 cup of barley

1/4 cup of great northern beans

6 cups of water

INSTRUCTIONS

1. Pour six cups of water in a large pot, add the beans and heat until its boiling. Reduce to medium heat after 5 minutes and let is simmer for 1 hour.

2. Add the chicken and onions and cook for 30 minutes, add the spices and taco seasoning. Cook further for 10 minutes.

3. Transfer everything in the in food processor and puree until smooth.

Nutrition per servings:

Protein: 13g

SOFT FOOD

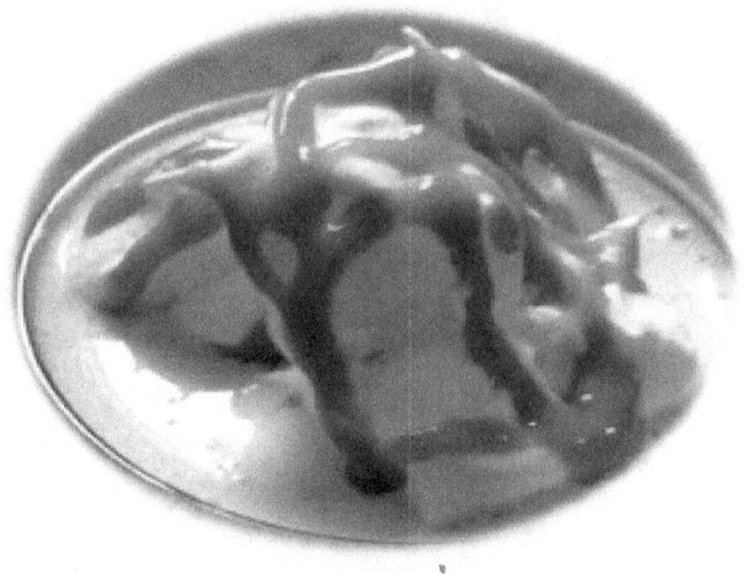

Richey's Baked Ricotta

Prep time: 5 minutes

Ready time: 30 minutes

Servings: Makes 1 pan

INGREDIENTS

1/2 cup shredded mozzarella cheese

8 ounces ricotta cheese

Salt & pepper

1 teaspoon Italian seasoning

1 large egg, beaten

1/2 cup marinara sauce

1 1/2 cup grated parmesan cheese

INSTRUCTIONS

1. In a mixing bowl, mix together the parmesan cheese, ricotta cheese, egg, seasonings. Place in an oven safe bowl. Pour mozzarella cheese and marinara over the top.

2. Place in the oven and bake for about 20-25 minutes at 450.

Nutrition per servings

Calories: 588kcal; Carbohydrates: 24g; Protein: 67g; Fat: 65g

Prep time: 10 minutes
Ready time: 30 minutes
Servings: 2

INGREDIENTS

6 ounces of frozen cauliflower rice
1/6 cup of asiago cheese shredded (or any cheese you prefer)
Optional: smoked paprika
1/6 cup of grated Parmesan
Salt and pepper, to taste
1/8 cup of shredded mild cheddar cheese
1/2 tbsp of butter
1/2 cup of milk
1/2 tsp of xanthan gum
1/6 cup of shredded sharp cheddar cheese

INSTRUCTIONS

1. Prepare the oven and heat-up to 350 F degrees.
2. Heat your frying pan over medium heat until it's hot. Place the butter in the heated pan until just melted. Swiftly whisk in the xanthan gum to form a paste. Whisk in the milk until no more lumps.
3. Cook the mixture for about 1-2 minutes, until mixture starts to thicken.
4. Add in the cheeses and mix until it starts to melt. Cook further for 5 to 7 minutes.
5. Mix the hot cheese mixture and bag of frozen cauliflower rice together in a bowl. Scoop the mix into a very small casserole dish or ramekins and bake, uncovered in the preheated oven, until cheese is done as desired, about 30 minutes.

Nutrition per servings
Calories: 241kcal; Carbohydrates: 19g; Protein: 14g; Fat: 14g

Prep time: 5 minutes

Ready time: 25-30 minutes

Servings: 3

INGREDIENTS

Two tbsp of Butter

Half cup of cheese

Half cup of milk

Three eggs

Cooked veggies (pureed)

INSTRUCTIONS

1. Crack the eggs open in a baking dish and beat together until smooth. Add milk, melted butter, cheese and add pureed veggies. (I love mushrooms and spinach)

2. Cook in the oven for 25-30 minutes at 375 degree.

Nutrition per servings.

Calories: 284kcal; Protein: 15g

Bacon Lemony Deviled Eggs

Prep time: 10 minutes
Ready time: 18 minutes
Servings: 6

INGREDIENTS

1/2 lemon zest
1 tbsp of chopped fresh chives
Freshly ground black pepper, to taste
Kosher salt, to taste
1/8 tsp of cayenne pepper
1 slices bacon, diced
1 tbsp of chopped fresh cilantro leaves
1/2 avocado, peel
3 large eggs
1/2 tbsp of freshly squeezed lemon juice

INSTRUCTIONS

1. Heat a large skillet over medium high heat. Add the diced bacon and cook about 6-8 minutes or until brown and crispy. Set aside on a plate lined with paper towel.
2. Cook the eggs in saucepan for few minutes, making sure the water is an inch above the eggs. Once it comes to a boil, cook for one minute more, cover the saucepan with a tight-fitted lid and remove saucepan from heat; let stand for 8-10 minutes. Drain.
3. Let eggs cool until you can handle without being hurt, peel and cut in half lengthwise, reserve the yolks.
4. Mash the avocado and yolks in a small bowl using a fork until it's chunky. Stir in lemon zest and lemon juice, cilantro, salt and pepper.
5. Pour the mixture into a pastry bag fitted with decorative tip then pipe the mixture into each egg halves. Top with bacon slices and garnish with cayenne pepper and chives, if desired.

Nutrition per servings
Calories: 131kcal; Carbohydrates: 2g; Protein: 5g; Fat: 11g

Prep time: 5 minutes

Ready time: 5 minutes

Servings: 2

INGREDIENTS

4 tbsp of salsa (such as Tostito's medium)

4 tbsp of plain fat-free Greek yogurt

2 tbsp of shredded Mexican blend cheese

2 oz of ground chicken or tofu or ground beef

2 whole eggs

Black pepper and salt to taste

2 egg whites

INSTRUCTIONS

1. Spray your griddle lightly using non-stick spray and heat over a medium heat.

2. In a mixing bowl, beat the eggs with egg whites together until well mixed. Pour half of the beaten eggs onto the pan and tilt around to allow the egg spread over the bottom. Cook for a minute or two, add black pepper and salt on top.

3. Lift the cooked egg with a spatula and cook the other side for about two minutes or until cooked. Transfer to a plate. Repeat with the remaining half.

4. Top with your choice of protein and Mexican cheese. Roll up from one end to the other to form egg-chilada. Add salsa and Greek yogurt on top.

Nutrition per servings:

Calories: 171kcal; Carbohydrates: 3g; Protein: 23g; Fat: 8g

Soft Baked Cheesy

Prep time: 6 minutes

Cook time: 30 minutes

Servings: 4

INGREDIENTS

1 cup of low-fat or fat-free cottage cheese

5-oz of frozen spinach (defroze and drained)

1 whole egg

1/4 cup of Parmesan cheese

Pinch of salt and pepper (optional)

Just a little minced garlic cloves (optional)

INSTRUCTIONS

1. Prepare the oven and heat-up to 350° F.

2. Mix the entire ingredients together in large bowl until well mixed.

3. Transfer the mixture evenly into a baking pan.

4. Bake in the oven at 350° F for 20-30 minutes. Remove and Let sit for 5 minutes before you serve.

Nutrition per servings

Calories: 78kcal; Carbohydrates: 2g; Protein: 11g; Fat: 3g

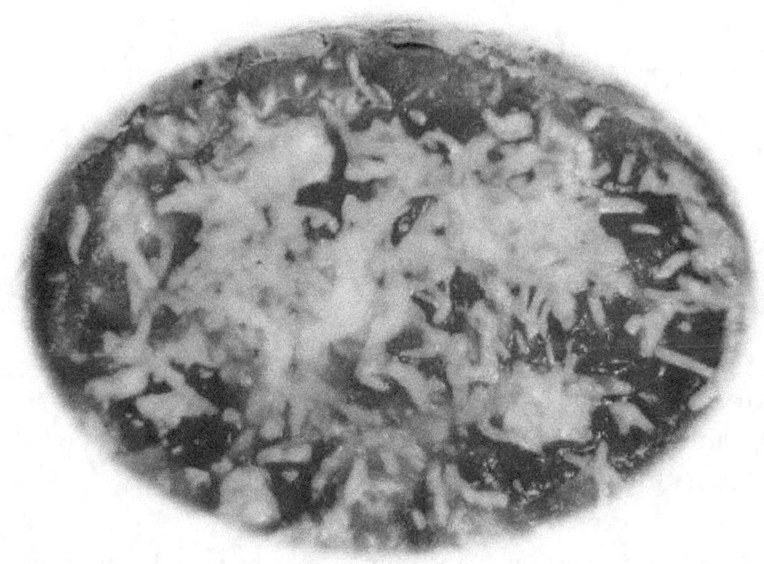

Prep time: 5 minutes
Freeze time: 4 hours
SERVINGS: 12
INGREDIENTS
2 cups of mixed berries or chopped fruits
1 cup of oats (instant or regular)
1 cup of milk 1% or skim
2 cup of Greek yogurt, plain, non-fat
INSTRUCTIONS
1. Whisk the Greek yogurt and milk in a mixing bowl and pour evenly into popsicle molds. Top each molds with few berries and evenly divide the oatmeal evenly among each of the molds.
2. Stick an ice cream stick into the center of each molds and transfer to the freezer. Let freeze for up to four hours before serving. Run the popsicle mound under lukewarm water until easy to remove.

Nutrition per servings:
Calories: 75kcal; Carbohydrates: 9.5g; Protein: 5g; Fat: 0.6

Prep time: 5 minutes

Ready time: 35 minutes

Servings: 8

INGREDIENTS

1/2 tsp of salt

2 cups of blueberries

2 cup of raspberries

4 cups of nonfat evaporated milk

1/2 tsp of nutmeg

2 cups of water

2 tsp of vanilla extract

8 tsp of sugar substitute

4 large eggs

INSTRUCTIONS

1. Heat the oven to 350 degrees F. Grease a 9 by 13 baking dish with nonstick spray.

2. Pour a cup of water into a 9 by 13" baking dish, set side.

3. Beat the eggs, vanilla, salt and sugar substitute together in a small bowl until well mixed; add the milk and stir until blended.

4. Mix the blueberries and raspberries together and evenly spread onto the base of the 8 by 8 pan; layer with the custard/egg mixture.

5. Set the 8-x-8 baking pan into the 9-by-13 inch pan. (This helps to prevent the custard from curdling.)

6. Place pan in the oven and bake for 35 minutes. To test if it's done, insert a knife into the center and if it comes out clean, it's done. Remove pan from oven and sprinkle top with nutmeg.

Nutrition per servings:

Calories: 178kcal; Carbohydrates: 21g; Protein: 13g; Fat: 3g

Prep time: 10 minutes

Cook time: 15 minutes

Servings: 2

INGREDIENTS

1/4 fresh lemon (juiced)

1/2 spring onion, coarsely chopped

1/2 tsp of butter

150 grams of white fish fillets

1 tsp of chopped dill

1/2 tsp of finely grated lemon rind

1/2 tsp of olive oil

Pea puree:

1/2 tsp of butter

1/2 spring onion (coarsely chopped)

125 grams of frozen baby peas

1/4 cup of hot chicken stock

INSTRUCTIONS

1. Prepare the oven and heat-up to 180 C.

2. Cut a piece of baking paper; large enough to wrap the fish fillet.

3. Place the fish in a large piece of baking paper, add butter, lemon rind and juice, half spring onion, olive oil and dill on top; season with salt and pepper.

4. Fold up the sides twice to seal and fold both ends in, then tuck in to seal.

5. Bake the fish in the oven for 10-15 minutes.

6. As the fish cooks, pour the stock into a medium saucepan, add the spring onion and peas; bring to a boil and cook for five minutes; drain. Reserve the liquid from cooking. Place the peas back to the pan. Add in the butter, and mix well using a stick blender, adding some of the reserved liquid if needed.

7. Serve the pea puree in serving plates, place the cooked fish on top and drizzle with the juices.

Nutrition per servings:
Calories: 614kcal; Carbohydrates: 5.5g; Protein: 19g; Fat: 4.5g

Quinoa Chicken Sausage Meatballs

Prep time: 10 minutes

Cook time: 18 minutes

Servings: 16 meatballs

INGREDIENTS

1/4 tsp of sea salt

1 tbsp of fresh oregano leaves

8 iceberg lettuce leaves

1/8 tsp of freshly ground black pepper

125 grams of chicken or turkey sausage, remove the casings

1/4 cup of feta cheese crumbles

1/2 cup of cooked and cooled quinoa (gotten from quarter cup dry)

1/4 red capsicum, remove the membranes and slice into strips

1 tbsp of fresh parsley leaves

1 garlic cloves

1/4 cup of shredded carrot

250 grams of extra-lean beef mince

Favorite choice of dressing

INSTRUCTIONS

1. Preheat your oven to 180 degrees C.

2. Place the carrot, red capsicum, garlic, oregano and parsley in a food processor and process until coarsely chopped.

3. In a medium mixing bowl, combine the chicken or turkey sausage, cooked quinoa, carrot mixture, ground beef, cheese, pepper and salt.

4. Mold the mixture into 16 meatballs using hands and place onto a parchment paper lined baking sheet.

5. Place in the oven and bake for 15 to 18 minutes at 180 degrees C or until golden brown and cooked through.

6. Spread a dollop of your favorite dressing over each lettuce leaf in the center. Top each with two meatballs.

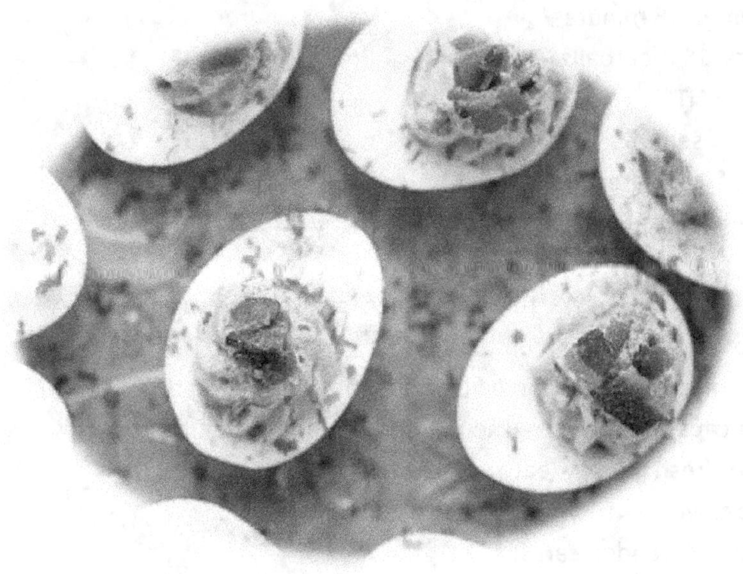

Prep time: 60 minutes
Cook time: 15 minutes
Servings: 2

INGREDIENTS

2 tsp of chili powder
1/4 tsp of salt
3/8 tsp of ground cumin
1 tsp of grated lemon rind
1/8 tsp of cinnamon
1/8 cup of pineapple juice
1 tbsp of brown sugar
2 (6 ounces each) salmon fillets
1 tbsp of fresh lemon juice

INSTRUCTIONS

1. Spray your baking dish with cooking spray. Heat-up your oven to 400 F.
2. Combine 1 tbsp lemon juice, pineapple juice and the salmon fillets in Ziploc bag.
3. Place in the refrigerator and marinate for 1 hour or so turning the salmon fillets periodically. Discard the marinade and set the salmon aside.
4. Combine the lemon rind, brown sugar, cinnamon, ground cumin, chili powder and salt in a mixing bowl; rub mixture over fish.
5. Place fish into the prepared baking dish. Bake at 400 F for 12-15 minutes. Serve with slices of lemon.

Nutrition per servings:
Calories: 225kcal; Carbohydrates: 7g; Protein: 34g; Fat: 6g

Prep time: 8 minutes
Cook time: 50 minutes
Servings: 3

INGREDIENTS

1/8 cup of low fat parmesan cheese
1/8 cup of pine nuts (Optional)
Greek Seasoning to taste (Penzey's is preferred)
Olive oil spray
3 large tomatoes, slice in half lengthways

INSTRUCTIONS

1. Prepare the oven and heat-up to 350º F.
2. Place the cut side of the tomato halves in a non-stick 8 by 8 inch pan. Spray the open side with olive oil spray and coat with pie nuts and cheese. Sprinkle with the seasoning to taste.
3. Place the pan in the oven and bake on middle rack of the oven for 50 minutes.

Nutrition per servings:
Calories: 73kcal; Carbohydrates: 4g; Protein: 3g; Fat: 5g

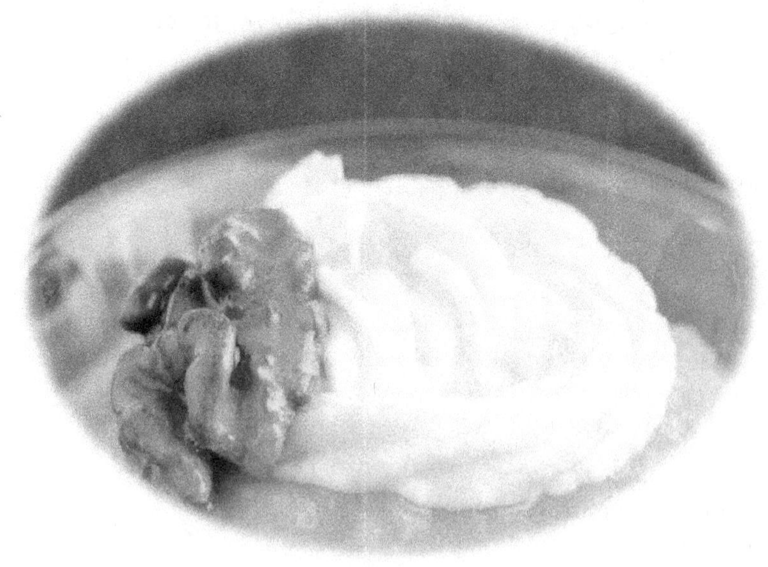

Tasty Pumpkin Pie Oatmeal

Prep time: 5 minutes

Cook time: 2 mutes

Servings: 2

INGREDIENTS

1 cup of 1% cottage cheese (no salt added)

2 tsp of Truvia baking blend

Dash of ground ginger

Dash of ground cloves

1/4 tsp of cinnamon

1 cup of pumpkin, canned

60 grams of old fashioned oats

INSTRUCTIONS

1. Combine all the ingredients in a heat-safe bowl with the exception of cottage cheese; microwave for 1 minute 30 seconds on high. Add the cottage cheese and stir.

Microwave for another 60 seconds on high. Allow to cool for a few minutes before serving.

Nutrition per servings:
Calories: 205kcal; Carbohydrates: 22g; Protein: 14g; Fat: 3g

No Bake Cheesecake Bowl

Prep time: 5 minutes
Ready time: 5 minutes
Servings: 3

INGREDIENTS

1/2 serving protein powder
8 ounces of cottage cheese
1/2 package of Sugar-Free Jell-O Instant Pudding and Pie Filling, Cheesecake Flavor
2 tbsp of fat-free milk
4 ounces of sugar-free cool whip

INSTRUCTIONS

1. Mix the entire ingredients in a food processor and blend until it's smooth. Chill in the refrigerator and serve. You can keep for at least two weeks in the refrigerator.

Nutrition per servings:
Protein: 11.7g

Cooked Fish With Garlic Lime

Prep time: 5 minutes

Ready time: 10 minutes

Servings: 2

INGREDIENTS

1 cloves garlic, smashed

1/2 tbsp of turmeric, grated

1/2 tbsp of grated fresh ginger

1 tbsp of olive oil

1/2 tbsp of tamari soy sauce

1 (200 grams) white fish fillets

Pinch of ground black pepper

1/2 bunch of coriander - leaves and stalk chopped finely

1/2 lime

INSTRUCTIONS

1. Combine together the garlic, ginger, lime juice, tamari soy sauce, olive oil and turmeric in a small bowl. Gently mix in the coriander root. Toss in the fish and stir to coat well.

2. Wrap the fish with foil or baking paper, then seal into little pocket to keep intact.

3. Steam the fish until it's cooked through, about 10 minutes; remove from the heat. Serve with vegetables or salad.

Fruity Cocoa Solace

Prep time: 5 minutes

Ready time: 10 minutes

Servings: 4

INGREDIENTS

1 tbsp of cornstarch

1/2 tsp of vanilla extract

1/8 to 1/4 tsp of almond or spearmint extract

1/2 cup of cold coffee

1/4 cup of sugar

1 cups of fresh cherries, strawberries or ripe apple

1/4 cup of unsweetened cocoa

INSTRUCTIONS

1. Whisk the cornstarch, cocoa, coffee and sugar over medium heat in a medium saucepan until bubbles stars to form and its thickened. Turn heat off and add the extracts.

2. Dip the fruit In chilled or warm sauce.

Nutrition per servings:

Calories: 79kcal; Carbohydrates: 17g; Protein: 3g; Fat: 1g

Basil, Tomato With Pasta Caprese

Prep time: 10 minutes

Ready time: 12 minutes

Servings: 4

INGREDIENTS

4 tbsp of extra-virgin olive oil

1/2 cup of fresh basil, julienned

2 tbsp of balsamic vinegar

4 oz of part-skim mozzarella, cubed

1/2 tsp of salt

2 pint grape tomatoes, quartered

4 oz of linguine pasta

4 tsp of olive oil

1/2 tsp of pepper

INSTRUCTIONS

1. Add water along with four tsp of olive oil in a medium saucepan over medium high heat. Add the pasta and cook according to package instructions. Drain and set aside for about 15 minutes.

2. Add the vinegar, tomatoes, olive oil; season with pepper and salt. Add the basil and mozzarella to the cooled pasta.

Nutrition per servings:

Calories: 371kcal; Carbohydrates: 24g; Protein: 12g; Fat: 23g

Prep time: 5 minutes
Ready time: 7 minutes
Servings: 8

INGREDIENTS

1/2 tsp of cumin
1/2 tsp of onion powder
1/2 tsp of chili powder
2/3 tsp of cilantro
Olive Oil spray
2 cup of vegetable broth
2 can of pinto beans drained and rinsed
1/2 tsp of garlic powder

INSTRUCTIONS

1. Lightly spray your sauté pan with olive oil cooking spray.
2. Pour in the drained pinto beans to the pan and cook about 1 to 2 minutes. Add the onion powder, broth, cumin, garlic powder and chili powder. Bring the mixture to a slow boil and cook until reduced by half.
3. Mash the pinto beans mixture until smooth. Garnish with cilantro, add shredded Mexican Cheese on top if you wish.

Nutrition per servings:
Calories: 85kcal; Carbohydrates: 19g; Protein: 5.9g; Fat: 0.8g

SOLID/REGULAR FOOD

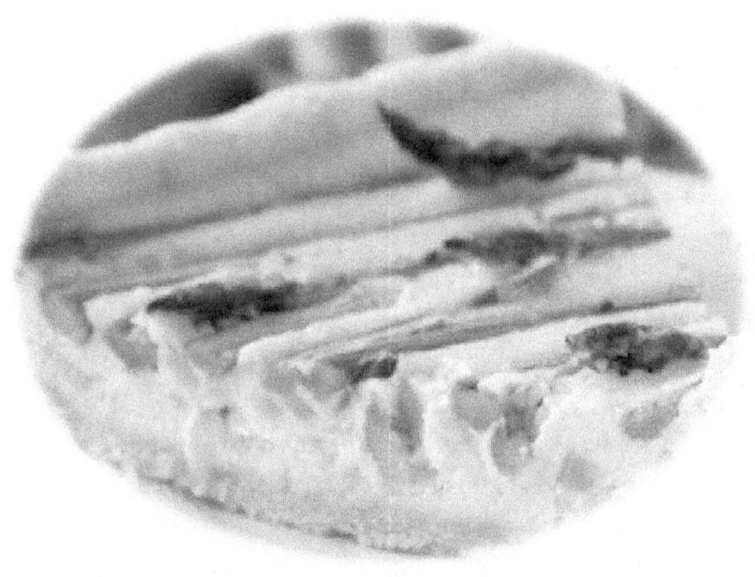

Crusty Butternut Squash Chicken Casserole

Prep time: 30 minutes

Ready time: 30 minutes

Servings: 8

INGREDIENTS

1 cup of frozen butternut squash

1/2 cup of whole wheat panko breadcrumbs

1/2 cup of shredded cheddar cheese

1 apple peeled and diced

1 lb of ground chicken

1/2 cup of low-fat milk

1 can of low-fat Cream of Chicken Soup

INSTRUCTIONS

1. Preheat the oven to 350 F.

2. Gently cook the ground chicken in a sauté pan over medium heat until it's cooked through. Pour in the low-fat milk of chicken soup; stir until everything is well mixed.

3. Cook the ground chicken mixture until sauce is starting to bring bubbles. Add the butternut squash and diced apple. Cook for about 10-15 minutes.

4. Evenly spread the chicken mixture onto your baking dish. Layer top with 1/2 cup of shredded cheddar cheese; layer with 1/2 cup of breadcrumbs.

5. Place baking dish in the oven and bake for 10 minutes or until cheese melts.

Nutrition per servings:

Calories: 150kcal; Carbohydrates: 7g; Protein: 12g; Fat: 7g

Turkey Berries Meatballs With Gruyere

Prep time: 5 minutes

Ready time: 20 minutes

Servings: 32 balls

INGREDIENTS

Turkey gravy to serve (homemade or prepared)

1/2 tsp of dried sage

1/4 tsp of black pepper

Pinch of salt

2/3 cup of dried cranberries no sugar added

2/3 cup of Gruyere shredded

2 eggs

2/3 cup of breadcrumbs plain

2 lb of lean ground turkey

INSTRUCTIONS

1. Prepare the oven and heat-up to 350 degrees F. Spray your baking pan with olive oil cooking spray.

2. Combine the cranberries, gruyere, turkey, breadcrumbs, sage, salt and pepper in a bowl.

3. Mold using your wet hands into balls, about 1 1/2-2 tbsp. measurement.

4. Transfer meatballs onto the baking pan and bake until meatball reach 165 degrees F, about 15-20 minutes. Serve with the turkey gravy.

Nutrition per servings: 3 meatballs per servings

Calories: 172kcal; Carbohydrates: 10g; Protein: 21g; Fat: 4.6g

Prep time: 10 minutes

Ready time: 30 minutes

Servings: 8

INGREDIENTS

2 yellow bell peppers, remove seed and cut into strips

2 medium yellow onion, slice into strips

2 red bell peppers, remove seed and cut into strips

4 tsp. minced garlic

1 lb. thin-cut steak cut into strips (Buy for pan frying)

2 tbsp of extra-virgin olive oil

Cayenne pepper

Salt and pepper to taste

2 tsp of coriander divided

2 tsp of chili pepper divided

2/3 cup of water

8 cup of frozen cauliflower rice

4 tbsp of tomato paste

2 tsp of cumin, divided

INSTRUCTIONS

1. Add the olive oil into hot frying pan. Sauté the onion, garlic and peppers over medium heat for about 5-7 minutes until softened.

2. Meanwhile, in a bowl, Add 1 tbsp of the cumin, place the steak strips, add half of coriander and half of chili pepper, salt and pepper.

3, Transfer the steak into your pan and sauté until it's browned. Add in the cauliflower rice and stir, cook for few minutes until it's thawed. Add the remaining spices and tomato paste. Add water if too thick.

4. Turn heat down to medium low and cover. Cook stirring constantly for about 10-15 minutes. Taste and adjust with the seasonings if needed.

5. Top with diced avocado, shredded cheese, jalapeno peppers.

Nutrition per servings: 3 meatballs per servings
Calories: 186kcal; Carbohydrates: 10g; Protein: 8g; Fat: 10g

Jolly Balsamic Pork Tenderloin

Prep time: 40 minutes

Ready time: 25 minutes

Servings: 8

INGREDIENTS

1 tsp of cracked black pepper

2 pound of pork tenderloin

2 tsp of olive oil

6 garlic cloves

5 tsp of coarse sea salt

4 tbsp of balsamic vinegar

INSTRUCTIONS

1. Blend the olive oil, black pepper, balsamic vinegar, garlic and salt in a bowl until its smooth; pour over pork. Set aside and marinate at least 30 minutes or overnight if you have enough time.

2. Prepare the oven and heat-up to 400 degrees F.

3. Brown the pork on both sides in a grill pan over medium heat.

4. Place browned pork in the oven and bake for about 20 minutes.

Nutrition per servings:

Carbohydrates: 3g; Protein: 23g; Fat: 4g

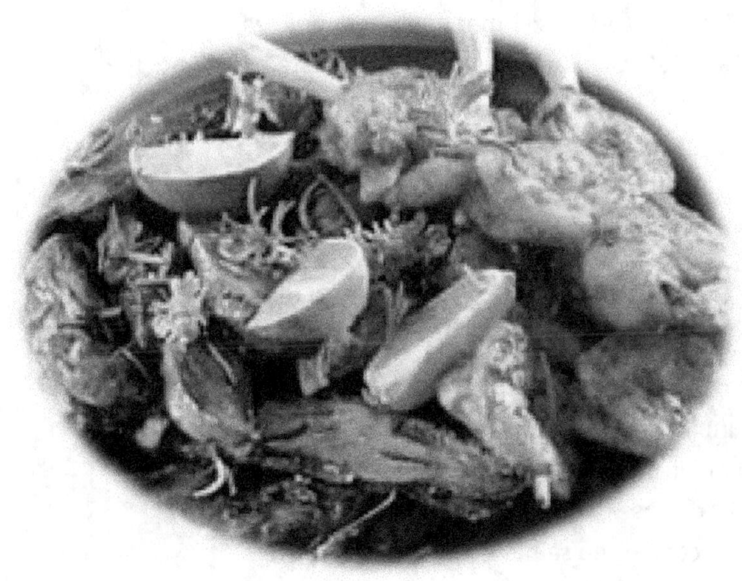

Easy Meatloaf With Sauce

Prep time: 10 minutes

Ready time: 45 minutes

Servings: 12

INGREDIENTS

1/2 cup of 2% mozzarella cheese, shredded

2 lightly beaten eggs

1/2 cup of onion, finely chopped

2 lb of lean ground beef

2 tsp Italian seasoning

1 cup of grated parmesan cheese, divided

1 cup of spaghetti sauce, divided

INSTRUCTIONS

1. Heat-up the oven to 375°F. Mix 1/2 spaghetti sauce, meat, 1/2 cup of shredded mozzarella cheese, grated parmesan cheese, egg, onion and seasoning.

2. Spread the meat mixture in a baking dish. Add the remaining 1/2 cup cheese and spaghetti sauce on top.

3. Place in the oven and bake until cooked through and the internal temperature reads 160°F, about 40 to 45 minutes.

Nutrition per servings:

Calories: 84kcal; Carbohydrates: 3g; Protein: 31g; Fat: 10g

Tomatoes Shrimp Basil

Prep time: 5 minutes

Ready time: 8 minutes

Servings: 8

INGREDIENTS

4 tbsp of fresh chopped basil

4 tbsp of grated parmesan cheese

4 tbsp of Light Italian Dressing

2 (14.5 oz each) can of Diced Tomatoes

2 pounds of medium frozen shrimp, thaw and remove tails

INSTRUCTIONS

1. Drop the shrimp in a large bowl and pour the Italian dressing over. Set aside.

2. Heat a non-stick skillet over medium heat and spray using cooking spray or olive oil. Toss in the shrimp and cook, stirring occasionally for about 5 minutes. Place the tomatoes; stir and cook further for 2-3 minutes.

3. Turn heat off and serve. Top with shaved parmesan cheese and grated parmesan cheese.

Nutrition per servings:

Carbohydrates: 5g; Protein: 30g; Fat: 1g

Cucumber Mayo Bites

Prep time: 5 minutes

Ready time: 10 minutes

INGREDIENTS

2 cooked chicken breast, diced into small squares

2 tsp of ground pepper

2 tsp of salt

1 cucumber sliced into circles

2/3 cup of thinly diced red onion

2/3 cup of light Mayonnaise

INSTRUCTIONS

1. Mix together the chicken breast, light mayonnaise, onions, pepper and salt in a bowl. Spoon 2 tbsp. of the mixture on top each slice of cucumber.

My Taco Beef Chili

Prep time: 10 minutes

Ready time: 15 minutes

Servings: 12

INGREDIENTS

2 packet of taco seasoning

30 oz, 2 cans of black beans, drained and rinsed

20 oz, 2 cans of diced green chiles and tomatoes

2 packet of ranch seasoning

2 pounds of 93% lean ground beef or turkey

INSTRUCTIONS

1. Pour the ground beef or turkey in a large stockpot, cook until brown; drain. Add the taco packets and ranch seasoning and stir until combined.

2. Stir in the black beans and tomatoes; reduce to low heat and simmer for about 10 minutes. If desired, serve with Greek Yogurt, canned jalapenos 2% shredded cheddar cheese

Nutrition per servings:
Carbohydrates: 9g; Protein: 26g; Fat: 8g

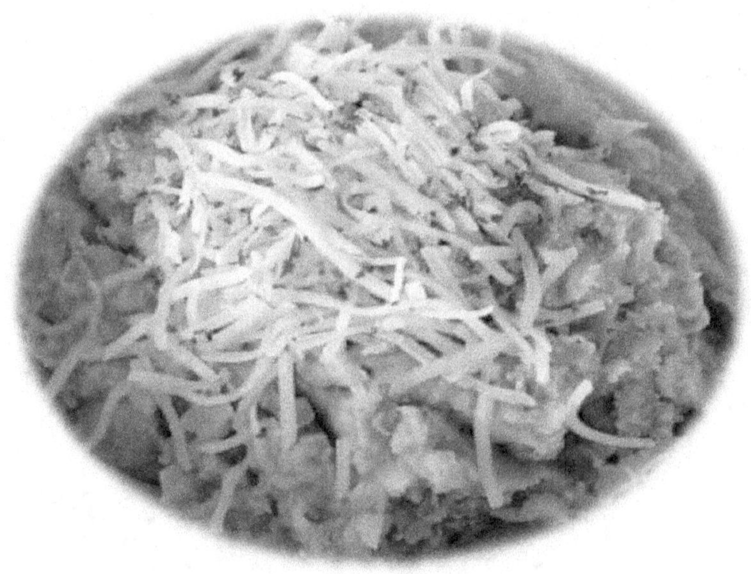

Cooked Prawn With Toasted Walnut Lime Juice

Prep time: 10 minutes

Servings: 2

INGREDIENTS

30 grams of crumbled Persian feta

60 grams of mixed leaf salad

15 grams of lightly toasted walnut halves

1/2 freshly squeezed lime juice

1/2 medium mango, peeled and cut into cubes

100 grams of cooked tiger prawns, peeled

100 grams of cherry tomatoes, halved

1/2 small avocado, peeled and cut into cubes

1/2 small finely sliced red capsicum

INSTRUCTIONS

1. Combine the mixed leaf salad, cherry tomatoes, avocado, capsicum, prawns, mango, walnuts and feta on a medium platter. Dress with the lime juice.

Nutrition per servings:

Calories: 880kcal; Carbohydrates: 112g; Protein: 14g; Fat: 10.5g

Shrimp Onion Serrano Ceviche

Ready time: 25 minutes
Servings: 8
INGREDIENTS
8 medium Italian or Roma tomatoes, diced
2 bunch of cilantro, stemmed and chopped finely
2 small finely chopped red onion
 (Optional) 3-4 serrano chili peppers, seeds and ribs removed, minced
Salt to taste
2 cup of lime juice
2 lb of medium raw shrimp
INSTRUCTIONS
1. Place the shrimp in a bowl, add the lime juice and stir to combine.
2. Cover with foil and let it marinate for 12 minutes or until color turns pink. If the shrimp stays too long, it will toughen. Add tomatoes, onions, cilantro and chili peppers. Stir gently to combine; Season with salt. Best serve cold.

Nutrition per servings:
Calories: 160kcal; Carbohydrates: 9g; Protein: g; Fat: 1g

Chicken Breast Tomato Caprese

Prep time: 20 minutes

Ready time: 10 minutes

Servings: 2

INGREDIENTS

2 (1-ounce) slices of fresh mozzarella cheese

1 tbsp of thinly sliced basil

1.5 tbsp of balsamic vinegar

Salt and pepper to taste

1/2 lb of skinless, boneless chicken breasts

2 (½-inch) thick slices of ripe tomato

1/2 tsp of dry Italian seasoning

1/2 tbsp of olive oil

INSTRUCTIONS

1. Preheat the grill for medium high heat.

2. Place the chicken breasts in a bowl, drizzle top with half tablespoon of olive oil and season with salt and pepper to taste. Sprinkle the seasoning over top.

3. Transfer the prepared chicken over to the grill and grill on each side for 3 to 5 minutes, or until it's done. Top with mozzarella cheese slice and cook further for one minute.

4. Once done, remove chicken from heat and set aside on a plate. Add thinly sliced basil, 1 slice of tomato on top, season with pepper to taste. Drizzle top with balsamic glaze to serve.

Nutrition per servings:

Calories: 230kcal; Carbohydrates: 4g; Protein: 33g; Fat: 9g

Black Bean Corn With Parsley Salad

Ready time: 40 minutes

Servings: 3

INGREDIENTS

1/2 tsp of lemon juice

Salt to taste

1/2 tsp of honey or brown sugar

1/2 tsp of garlic, minced

1/8 tsp of ground black pepper

1 tbsp of olive oil

1 tbsp of red onion, minced

1/2 cup of corn, whole kernel

1/8 cup of parsley, chopped fresh

1 (15-oz) can of black beans, rinsed and drained

1/8 cup of balsamic vinegar

INSTRUCTIONS

1. In a mixing bowl, mix the black beans, fresh corn, fresh parsley and red onion together until well mixed.

2. In a different mixing bowl, blend together the olive oil, honey, balsamic vinegar, garlic, lemon juice, salt and pepper.

3. Pour the balsamic vinegar mixture on top corn/black beans mixture. Marinade for about 30 minutes before serving.

Nutrition per servings:

Calories: 160kcal; Carbohydrates: 16g; Protein: 6g; Fat: 5g

Seasoned Chicken Applesauce

Prep time: 10 minutes

Cook time: 1 hour

Servings: 4

INGREDIENTS

Salt and pepper to taste

1/4 cup of powdered peanuts

1/2 jar (7.5 oz) of unsweetened applesauce

1 1/4 lbs of chicken pieces

1 tbsp of Splenda brown sugar, unpacked

1/8 cup of yellow mustard

INSTRUCTIONS

1. Cook the chicken pieces in a sauté pan until almost fully cooked. Add in the mustard, applesauce, powdered peanuts and brown sugar. Stir well.

2. Simmer for about 40 minutes over medium heat until internal temperature reaches 165ºF.

Nutrition per servings: 2 tablespoons

Calories: 50kcal; Carbohydrates: 11g; Protein: 3g; Fat: 2g

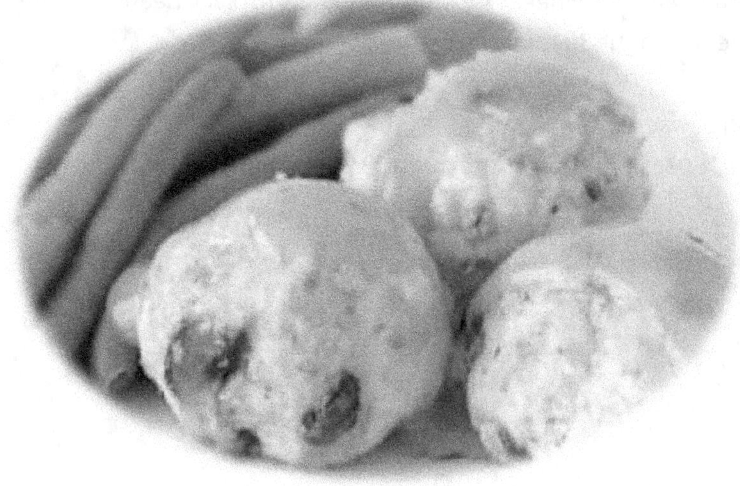

Veggie Peanut Bean Chili

Prep time: 10 minutes

Cook time: 35 minutes

Servings: 5 – 6

INGREDIENTS

1 tbsp of chili powder

1/2 can (7.5 ounce) tomato sauce

1 4 ounce can diced tomato

1/3 cup of powdered peanuts

1 cup of vegetable broth

8 ounce can of black beans, drained and rinsed

1/8 tsp of dried oregano

1/2 tbsp of peanut oil (or canola oil)

1/2 tsp of chipotle chili pepper (optional)

1 cloves garlic, minced

1/2 cup of chopped onion

8 ounce can of white beans, drained and rinsed

INSTRUCTIONS

1. Sauté the garlic and onion in a Dutch oven over medium high heat for about 3 – 4 minutes or until soften. Stir in oregano, chili powder, salt and pepper; Sauté until fragrant, about 2 minutes.

2. Add the powdered peanuts, beans, tomato sauce, tomatoes, and broth, bring to a boil. Turn heat down and let it simmer for 30 minutes.

Nutrition per servings: 1/2 cup

Calories: 125kcal; Carbohydrates: 10g; Protein: 8g; Fat: 2.5g

Prep time: 5 minutes

Cook time: 5 minutes

Servings: 2

INGREDIENTS

1 tbsp of powdered peanuts

1/2 cup frozen mixed berry blend

2 large egg whites

1/4 cup of instant oatmeal

1/4 cup of low-fat cottage cheese

INSTRUCTIONS

1. Whisk the cottage cheese, powdered peanuts, oatmeal and egg whites in a blender and process until mixture is well blended. Transfer into a small bowl and gently fold in berry blend.

2. Spray the frying pan with cooking spray; Scoop about 1/4 cup of the batter into the skillet and cook, flipping once it starts to bubble on top.

Nutrition per servings:

Calories: 90kcal; Carbohydrates: 7.5g; Protein: 10g; Fat: 1.5g

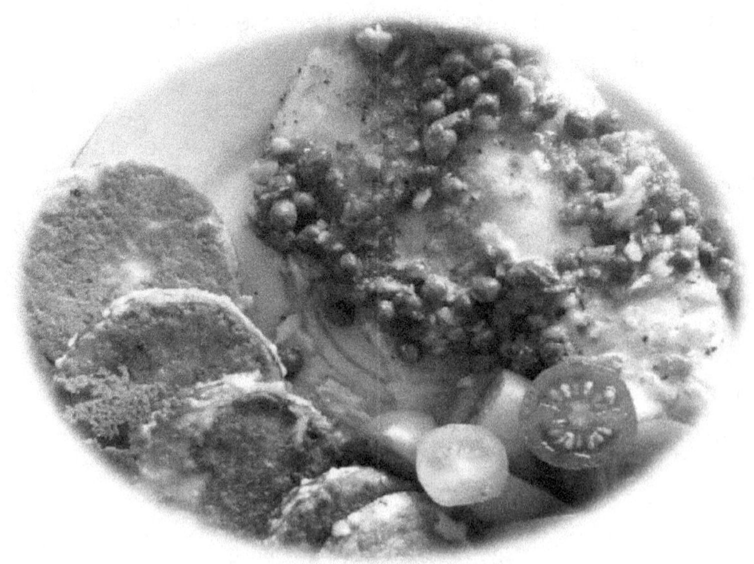

Pumpkin Protein Ricotta Pie

Prep time: 10 minutes

Cook time: 40 minutes

Servings: 6

INGREDIENTS

1 scoops of 100% Unflavored Whey Protein Isolate

1/2 tsp of ground nutmeg

1/2 tsp of ground cinnamon

1/4 tsp of salt

1 oz package pecan halves

1 cup of can of no salt added 100% pure pumpkin puree

1/6 cup of Truvia for Baking or Splenda Sugar Blend

1/2 cup of milk, nonfat (skim milk)

1 egg, large

1/2 cup of ricotta cheese, part skim

INSTRUCTIONS

1. Preheat the oven to 350ºF. Spray your pie dish along with two small ramekins using non-stick cooking spray.

2. Whisk 1/4 cup of milk, egg and ricotta cheese in a bowl until smooth and well combined. Add in the remaining ingredients into the bowl and process until mixture is smooth.

3. Add the mixture into the prepared dish, add pecans over top.

4. Place in the heated oven and bake until its cooked, double in size and middle is set, about 40 – 45 minutes. If the pie is browning at the top too quickly, reduce to 325º degrees F and cook until its set. Let cool about an hour before cutting into 12 pieces.

Nutrition per servings: 1 slice
Calories: 105kcal; Carbohydrates: 8g; Protein: 6g; Fat: 3.5g

Tuna Lettuce Sandwiches

Prep time: 5 minutes
Ready time: 10 minutes
Servings: 6
INGREDIENTS
1/2 cup of low-fat vanilla yogurt
12 whole wheat bread slices
1 tsp of honey
2 tsp of mustard
6 lettuces leaves
2 apples, peel and chop into small pieces
2 (13 ounces total) can of tuna, packed in water, drained
INSTRUCTIONS
1. Add the apple slices, tuna, mustard, honey and yogurt in a bowl; stir everything together.
2. Arrange the sliced bread on a flat plate and spread half cup of the tuna mix over each slices.
3. Add one lettuce leaf on top each and layer with another slice of bread.

Nutrition per servings:
Calories: 250kcal; Carbohydrates: 25g; Protein: 23g; Fat: 2.5g

Prep time: 20 minutes

Cook time: 15 minutes

Servings: 2

INGREDIENTS

1/2 tsp of mustard seeds

1.5 cm piece of ginger, peeled and chopped

1/2 tsp of cumin

1 x 150 grams of skinless chicken breast

1/2 cup of chopped spinach

1 cloves garlic, peeled and chopped

1/2 tsp of curry powder

1/2 small cauliflower, cut into flowerets

1/2 tsp of turmeric

1/2 lemon, divided

3 tbsp of low fat natural Greek yoghurt, divided

1/2 tbsp of balsamic vinegar

1/4 bunch of mint

INSTRUCTIONS

1. Prepare the oven and heat-up to 200°C

2. Add 1.5 tbsp yoghurt, half of the lemon juice, mint leaves, and dash of water in a blender and blend until smooth; then refrigerate until ready to use.

3. Add remaining half of the lemon juice and yoghurt into blender, add the balsamic, curry powder, turmeric, ginger and garlic; blend until you have a smooth marinade.

4. Score the chicken breasts lightly on the surface and coat in the marinade. Allow to rest for few minutes.

5. Remove coated chicken breast from the marinade and transfer into your baking tray and sprinkle with mustard seeds and the cumin. Bake until chicken is done, about 10-15 minutes.

6. Add the cauliflower in a food processor and blend until mixture has rice like texture. Cook for 3 minutes in a microwave vegetable steamer.
7. Serve cauliflower in two serving bowls and add chicken and chopped spinach on top. Spread the mint dressing on top.

Nutrition per servings:
Calories: 445kcal; Carbohydrates: 1.9g; Protein: 17g; Fat: 1.3g

Seasoned Meatballs With Hommus Dip

Prep time: 10 minutes
Cook time: 10 minutes
Servings: 2
INGREDIENTS
1/2 crushed garlic clove
1/2 lemon Juice
40 grams of hommus
1/2 tsp of olive oil
1/2 tsp of Harissa spice mix
1/2 small grated zucchini, drained
1/2 tsp of sweet paprika
1/2 small egg
1/4 cup of flat-leaf parsley leaves, coarsely chopped
1 tbsp of whole meal breadcrumbs
100 grams of lean pork mince
INSTRUCTIONS
1. Place the egg, grated zucchini, chopped parsley, breadcrumbs, pork mince, paprika, spice mix and garlic; season with black pepper and salt In a small bowl,. Mix until well blended. Roll mixture into four meatballs.
2. Transfer the meatballs into a plate and press down slightly with a fork. Cover and refrigerate for about 10 minutes.

3. Add together the hommus, 1 tbsp. warm water and lemon juice in a small bowl until well mixed.

4. In a non-stick frying pan, heat the oil over medium heat. Place the meatballs and cook for about 3 minutes per side. Serve the meatballs with hommus dip.

Nutrition per servings:

Calories: 650kcal; Carbohydrates: 5g; Protein: 10.8g; Fat: 8.8g

Salmon With Cauliflower Pine Nuts Mixture

Prep time: 5 minutes

Cook time: 15 minutes

Servings: 2

INGREDIENTS

1/4 cup of frozen peas

1 tbsp of chopped fresh parsley

1/2 tsp of olive oil

1/2 lemon juice and grated zest

1 (125 grams) of skinless salmon fillets

1/8 cup of toasted pine nuts

1/2 small cauliflower cut into florets

INSTRUCTIONS

1. Heat-up the oven to 356 degrees F. Line your baking tray with baking paper.

2. Arrange the salmon fillets on the prepared tray.

3. Place tray in the oven and bake until cooked through, about 10-15 minutes.

4. Pulse the cauliflower in a food processor into couscous like texture.

5. Place the peas and cauliflower in a heat-proof dish and cover; microwave for 3 minutes.

6. In a mixing bowl, Combine together the olive oil, pine nuts, parsley, lemon juice and zest and mix well

7. Serve the cooked salmon fillets in 2 serving dishes along with the cauliflower mixture.

Nutrition per servings:

Calories: 677kcal; Carbohydrates: 113g; Protein: 14g; Fat: 10g

Rice Paper Rolls Wraps

Prep time: 10 minutes

Servings: 2

INGREDIENTS

2 finely sliced spring onion

8 tsp of sweet chilli sauce

14 mint leaves

1 cup of grated carrot

8 rice paper sheets

240 grams of cooked chicken breast

1/2 cup of finely sliced cucumber and capsicum

1/2 cup of bean shoots

1/2 cup of shredded cabbage or lettuce leaves

INSTRUCTIONS

1. Drop all the rice paper into a pot of boiling water and leave to soak for 1 minute.

2. Remove and set the rice paper over a clean bread board, add 1/4 vegetables, 30 grams of the chicken, 2 mint leaves and 1 teaspoon of sweet chilli sauce.

3. Roll the rice paper roll up and transfer onto a plate. Repeat with remaining rice paper rolls.

Nutrition per servings:

Calories: 413kcal; Carbohydrates: 6.2g; Protein: 18g; Fat: 1.6g

Brown Rice With Black Bean Pork Verde Stew

Prep time: 15 minutes
Cook time: 55 minutes
Servings: 8

INGREDIENTS

(Optional) 2 tsp of crushed red pepper flakes
2 (14.5 ounces each) can of black beans, no salt added, drained &
rinsed
2 (14.5 ounces each) can of diced tomatoes in juice (no salt added)
2 (14 ounces each) can of chicken broth (no salt added)
2 packet Goya Sazon with coriander & annatto (or similar seasoning
packet)
2 tsp of ground cumin
4 cans of chipotle peppers in adobo sauce, minced + 2 tsp of adobo
sauce
5 garlic cloves
2 1/2 cup of chopped onions
2 lbs of pork loin or tenderloin, trimmed of visible fat and cut into 1
inch cubes
4 tsp of extra-virgin olive oil

INSTRUCTIONS

1. Heat the olive oil in large pot over medium high heat.Add the pork
and cook for 4-6 minutes, stirring periodically until browned.
2. Add the garlic and onion and cook further for 2-3 minutes or until
onion starts to soften. Add the cumin, chipotle peppers in adobo sauce
and the seasoning packet; mix well. Add the chicken broth, beans,
tomatoes and red pepper flakes (optional). Stir to combine. Bring
mixture to a boil then turn heat down to low.
3. Cover pot with a lid and let it simmer on low heat for 45 to 60
minutes or until the port is cooked. Serve stew over brown rice.

Nutrition per servings:
Calories: 308kcal; Carbohydrates: 19g; Protein: 33g; Fat: 7g

Prep time: 10 minutes

Cook time: 8 minutes

Servings: 2

INGREDIENTS

1/2 cup of sliced mushrooms

2 low-carb whole wheat flour tortilla

2 (1.5 ounces total) wedge of Swiss cheese (Laughing Cow Original light)

(Optional) 4 tsp of sliced pickled hot chili peppers

1/2 lb of skinless, boneless chicken breast, trimmed of visible fat

½ cup of sliced green pepper

1/2 cup of chopped onions

INSTRUCTIONS

1. Flatten the chicken breast by pounding into 1/4" thin on a cutting board, and slice thinly into strips.

2. Spray a skillet with cooking spray and place the pan over medium high heat. Add in the chopped onion with the chicken and cook until chicken is cooked through, about 5 minutes.

3. Add in the mushrooms slices and green peppers slices and cook for additional 2-3 minutes until mushrooms and peppers are tender.

4. Place each tortilla between two pieces of damp paper towels. Place in the microwave for 20 seconds.

5. Remove and place each warm tortilla on 2 flat platters and spread the cheese on top evenly.

6. Top with mushrooms, chicken, onions and peppers. Top with chili peppers if needed. Wrap tortilla from the sides. Serve immediately.

Nutrition per servings:

Calories: 264kcal; Carbohydrates: 13g; Protein: 33g; Fat: 6g

Spinach Onion Frittata

Prep time: 10 minutes
Cook time: 40 minutes
Servings: 12

INGREDIENTS

4 whole eggs
1/4 tsp of salt
1/2 tsp of cayenne pepper
2/3 cup of reduced-fat cottage cheese
1/4 tsp of nutmeg
4 tsp of vegetable oil
3 cups of shredded reduced-fat cheddar cheese
2 (20 oz total) package of chopped spinach, (frozen) thawed and drained
2 medium onions, chopped (if tolerated)
8 egg whites
9-by 13 pie pan

INSTRUCTIONS

1. Prepare the oven and heat to 375 F. Spray your pan with vegetable oil spray.
2. Heat the vegetable oil in a medium skillet over medium high heat. Add in the onion and cook until it's tender, about 5 minutes. Toss in the spinach and cook further for 3 minutes, keep aside. Sprinkle your pan with cheese and top with onion/spinach mixture.
3. Beat the whole eggs plus egg whites, cayenne pepper, cottage cheese, nutmeg and salt in a medium bowl.
4. Spread mixture over cheese and onion/spinach mixture in the pie pan.
5. Place pan in the oven and bake until just set, about 30 to 35 minutes or. Let cool for 5 minutes before cutting into wedges.

Nutrition per servings:
Calories: 162kcal; Carbohydrates: 6g; Protein: 16g; Fat: 8g

Prep time: 10 minutes

Cook time: 6 minutes

Servings: 4

INGREDIENTS

1/2 tsp of ground celery seeds

Salt to taste

1/2 tsp of ground black pepper

2 2/3 tbsp of chopped parsley

4 tsp of olive oil

6 tbsp of yellow cornmeal

16 oz of rainbow trout fillets, clean and remove all bones, pat dry

INSTRUCTIONS

1. In a clean medium mixing bowl, mix the cornmeal, celery seed, chopped parsley salt and pepper making sure it's well mixed.

2. Dip the fish in cornmeal mixture, making sure it's well coated.

3. In non-stick skillet, heat the olive oil and cook the fish in the hot skillet for about 2 to 3 minutes per side until crispy, brown and flake easy with a fork.

Nutrition per servings:

Calories: 240kcal; Carbohydrates: 7g; Protein: 25g; Fat: 10g

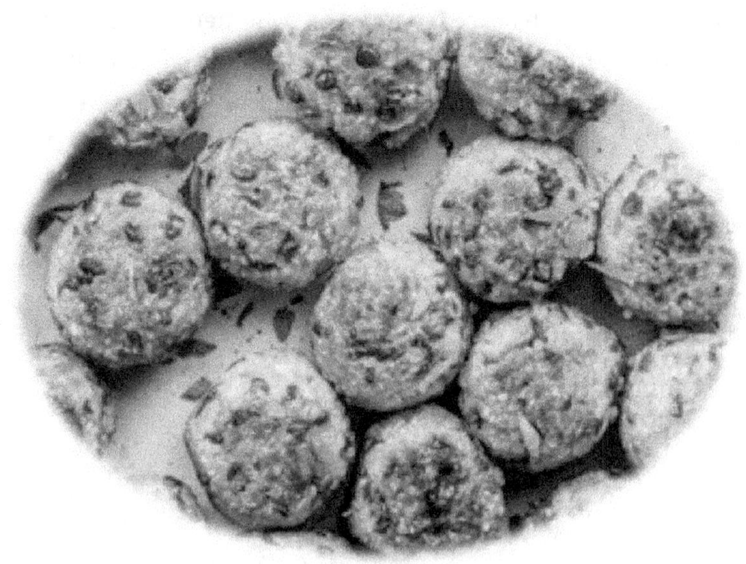

Black Bean Pumpkin Puree Soup

Prep time: 10 minutes

Cook time: 25 minutes

Servings: 3 (about 1 cup each)

INGREDIENTS

1/4 tsp of black pepper

1 cups of beef broth

1/2 cup of canned diced tomatoes

1 (15 ounce) cans of black beans, rinsed and drained

8 ounce can of pumpkin puree

1/2 tsp of chili powder

1/4-pound ground meat, optional

2 minced garlic cloves

1/2 medium chopped onion

1 tbsp of olive oil

Greek yogurt for added protein

1/2 tbsp of ground cumin

INSTRUCTIONS

1. In a stainless steel soup kettle, heat the oil over medium heat; add the garlic, onions, garlic, chili powder, ground cumin, and pepper, and sauté until soft. Stir in pumpkin, black beans, broth, ground meat, tomatoes and Greek yogurt.

2. Simmer uncovered for about 25 minutes, stirring occasionally until soup is thick. Puree the mixture using hand held blender until smooth or serve as it is.

Nutrition per servings:
Calories: 290kcal; Carbohydrates: 32g; Protein: 15g; Fat: 6g

Baked Pork Tenderloin

Prep time: 10 minutes
Cook time: 30-40 minutes
Servings: 4

INGREDIENTS

1/2 tbsp of dry mustard
2 garlic cloves minced
1/2 tbsp of ginger
1 lbs of pork tenderloin
1 tbsp of rice vinegar
1/6 cup of light soy sauce
1 tbsp of lemon juice
1 tbsp of Worcestershire sauce
1/6 cup of brown sugar
¾ tsp of pepper

INSTRUCTIONS

1. Pour the marinade ingredients into a sealable plastic bag and mix everything together.
2. Place the tenderloin into the bag and rub through with your hands.
3. Place bag in the refrigerator overnight to allow flavor mend.

4. Bake in the oven at 375º F degrees for 30-40 minutes or use your slow cooker on low for 4-6 hours.

Nutrition per servings:

Calories: 256kcal; Carbohydrates: 9g; Protein: 34g; Fat: 9g

Chicken Easy Bakes Greek Yogurt

Prep time: 15 minutes

Cook time: 45 minutes

Servings: 8

INGREDIENTS

2 tsp of garlic powder

1 tsp of pepper

3 tsp of seasoning salt

8 (4 ounces each) skinless, boneless chicken breasts

1 cup of grated Parmesan cheese

2 cup of plain Greek yogurt

INSTRUCTIONS

1. Prepare the oven and heat-up to 375 degrees F. Line your baking tray with foil and then spray with non-stick cooking spray.

2. In a clean mixing bowl, combine the grated Parmesan cheese, Greek yogurt, and seasonings.

3. Dip each chicken breast in the cheese/yogurt mixture until well coated and transfer onto the prepared baking sheet.

4. Place baking sheet in the oven and bake 375 degrees F for 45 minutes.

Nutrition per servings:

Calories: 266kcal; Carbohydrates: 3g; Protein: 46g; Fat: 4g

Prep time: 5 minutes

Cook time: 5 minutes

Servings: 8 pancakes

INGREDIENTS

5-6 eggs, lightly beaten

1 tbsp of canola oil

2 cup of low-fat cottage cheese

1 tsp of baking soda

2/3 cup of all-purpose flour

INSTRUCTIONS

1. Whisk together the flour and baking soda in a small bowl.

2. In another mixing bowl, combine together the remaining ingredients.

3. Combine the dry mixture into wet mixture and mix until just combined.

4. Place a large frying pan over medium heat, lightly spray with non-stick spray.

5. Scoop 1/8 of the mixture into the skillet and cook until it starts to bubble on the surface. Turn and cook until other side is brown. Serve with any low calorie syrup of your choice

Nutrition per servings:

Calories: 152kcal; Carbohydrates: 10g; Protein: 13g; Fat: 7g

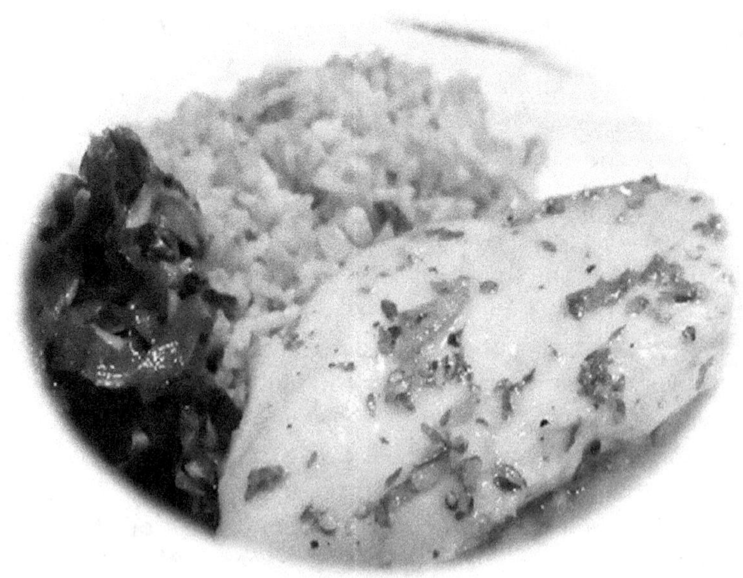

Broccoli Water Chestnuts Beef Stir Fry

Prep time: 15 minutes

Cook time: 15 minutes

Servings: 3

INGREDIENTS

1.5 oz of broccoli florets

1.5 tbsp of soy sauce

1 medium stalks of bok choy, cut into ½-inch slices

1/4 cup of instant brown rice

1/4 medium green, yellow or red bell pepper, cut into strips

4-oz can of sliced water chestnuts

1/8 tsp of crushed red pepper flakes

1/2 tbsp of cornstarch

1 ounce cup of hoisin sauce

0.5 lb of flank steak (cut into ¼-inch strips)

1 medium garlic cloves

1 tsp of ground ginger

1/2 tsp of canola oil

3 oz beef broth (fat free)

INSTRUCTIONS

1. Add the steak in a mixing bowl with ginger and garlic mix well and set aside.
2. Prepare the instant brown rice just as instructed in package directions.
3. Combine broth, cornstarch, soy sauce and hoisin sauce in a bowl. Stir until well combined and dissolved.
4. Heat the oil in a skillet over medium-high heat until it's hot, add red pepper flakes. Add the steak and cook stirring constantly for 4-5 minutes or until steak is browned. Set aside.
5. Add the carrot, bell pepper and broccoli into pan. Cook for 2-3 minutes over medium-high heat; Stir. (Add in 1 tbsp. water to the mixture if it's becoming too dry)
6. Stir in the water chestnuts and bok choy. Cook further for 1-2 minutes, stirring constantly or until its tender-crisp.
7. Create a hole in middle of the pan and pour in the broth.
Cook for additional 1 or 2 minutes, stirring constantly until broth thickens.
Add the beef and mix. Cook for few minutes until warm through. Serve over rice.

Nutrition per servings:
Calories: 275kcal; Carbohydrates: 21g; Protein: 17g; Fat: 8g

Cheese Turkey Bacon Muffin

Prep time: 10 minutes

Cook time: 20-25 minutes

Servings: 6

INGREDIENTS

1/4 cup of 1% milk

1/8 tsp of pepper

1/8 tsp of salt

1/8 tsp of Italian seasoning

3 large eggs

3/8 cup of shredded low fat Monterey jack or Swiss cheese

6 slices of pre-cooked turkey bacon (sliced 1/3)

INSTRUCTIONS

1. Prepare the oven and heat oven to 350º F. Spray 6 muffin tin using cooking spray.

2. To the base of each muffin tin, arrange 3 bacon slices.

3. Mix together the remaining ingredient (reserving 1/8 cup of the shredded cheese) in a separate bowl until well blended.

4. Pour 1/4 cup of the egg mixture into each muffin cup. Sprinkle top with the reserved 1/8 cup of cheese.

5. Place in the oven and bake until eggs are set, about 20-25 minutes.

Nutrition per servings:

Calories: 98kcal; Carbohydrates: 1g; Protein: 8g; Fat: 7g

Chicken Spinach/Cheese Blaze

Prep time: 15 minutes
Cook time: 40 minutes
Servings: 8
INGREDIENTS
Toothpicks
4 tsp of olive oil
2 tbsp of bread crumbs
4 tbsp of Cajun seasoning
2 lb of skinless, boneless chicken breasts (32 oz)
2 cups of frozen or fresh cooked spinach (thawed and drained if frozen)
6 ounces of Shredded pepper jack cheese (reduced fat)
INSTRUCTIONS
1. Prepare the oven and heat up to 350º F. Line your baking sheet with tin foil.
2. Flatten the chicken breast by pounding into 1/4" thin on a cutting board.
3. Blend the spinach, pepper jack cheese, pepper and salt in a medium bowl.
4. In a small bowl, combine together the breadcrumbs and Cajun seasoning until well combined.
5. Pour about a quarter cup of spinach/cheese mix over each chicken breast. Roll up tightly and hold the ends together with toothpicks. Brush all through with the olive oil and then sprinkle with the breadcrumbs mixture. If you have any remaining spinach/cheese mix, you may sprinkle over the chicken if you desire.
6. Place the seam-side of the chicken breast up over the prepared baking sheet.
7. Place baking sheet in the oven and bake until chicken is cooked, about 35 to 40 minutes.
8. Don't forget to remove all the toothpicks before you serve.

Nutrition per servings:
Calories: 241kcal; Carbohydrates: 1g; Protein: 32g; Fat: 9.7g

Chicken Carrots In Slow Cooker

Prep time: 10 minutes

Cook time: 4 hours

Servings: 6

INGREDIENTS

2 cup of light coconut milk

1 red bell pepper, cut into strips

1 tbsp of water

1 tbsp of corn starch

3 cup of cauliflower rice

1 tsp of garlic minced

3 tbsp of curry powder

1 cup of frozen peas

1 cup of low-sodium chicken broth

1 pounds of skinless, boneless chicken thighs

1 large carrot diced

1 medium yellow onion, cut into slices

1/4 tsp of each salt and pepper

INSTRUCTIONS

1. Place the chicken in a flat plate and Sprinkle with salt and pepper.

2. Transfer the chicken in a slow cooker along with the carrots, bell pepper, peas, curry powder, garlic and onion. Add the coconut milk and chicken broth and cook for 4 hours on low.

3. Remove cooked chicken from cooker onto a plate and gently shred.

4. Add water to a small mixing bowl, add the cornstarch and blend well until a paste forms.

5. Pour the cornstarch mix into the slow cooker and stir. Cook for about 10 minutes, and then place back the chicken. Cook further for an hour. Serve hot across cauliflower rice.

Nutrition per servings:
Calories: 330kcal; Carbohydrates: 9g; Protein: 23g; Fat: 19g

Prep time: 10 minutes

Cook time: 15 minutes

Servings: 4

INGREDIENTS

For the Tilapia

1 tbsp of butter

2 tsp of garlic minced

2 large lemons, juiced

1/2 cup of Champagne vinegar (or white cooking wine)

2 tbsp of capers

2 tbsp of all-purpose flour (or cornstarch)

2 tbsp of extra-virgin olive oil

Salt and pepper to taste

4 tilapia filets thawed if frozen

For the Parmesan crusted zucchini

Non-stick cooking spray

4 whole eggs

1 cup of grated Parmesan cheese

2 medium zucchini cut 1/4 inch thick rounds

INSTRUCTIONS

Make the Tiliapia

1. Generously spray a hot frying pan with non-stick spray over medium heat.

2. Season each tilapia filets all over with pepper and salt. Place in the pan and cook on each side for about 2 minutes. Remove and set aside.

3. Reduce to low heat, add the butter and flour to the pan; whisk until it simmering and starting to thicken. Add the lemon juice, Champagne vinegar and garlic, whisking for about 2-3 minutes.

4. Add in the capers and cook for additional 1-2 minutes. Taste and adjust with either 2 teaspoon of milk or butter. This will help calm it down if it makes you pucker. Spread sauce over fish to serve.

Make the zucchini

5. Place the eggs and cheese in different bowls.

6. Dredge each round of zucchini in the bowl of cheese, then dip in the egg bowl, dip inside the cheese again.

7. Generously spray hot frying pan with non-stick spray over medium heat. Cook the zuchinni in hot pan for about 2-3 minutes on both sides. Let it cook for more than half of the total time before flipping to allow the crust stick.

Transfer the zucchini and let drain on a paper towel before serving.

Best Zucchini Ravioli

Prep time: 15 minutes

Cook time: 30 minutes

Servings: 2

INGREDIENTS

1 cup of part-skim ricotta cheese

Optional: Additional Italian-blend shredded cheese

1/2 tsp of Italian seasoning

1/4 cup of grated parmesan cheese

1 medium zucchini, slice in 1/8 inch thick strips, length-wise

1/2 tbsp of tomato paste

1/4 tsp of cinnamon

1/2 small sliced onions

½ (7.5 ounces) can of pumpkin puree (different from pumpkin pie filling)

Salt and pepper, to taste

1/2 pounds of lean ground turkey

1/4 tsp. nutmeg

1/2 minced garlic clove

INSTRUCTIONS

1. Prepare the oven and heat-up to 350 F.

2. Generously spray hot frying pan with non-stick spray over medium heat. Sauté the onions in the hot skillet for 1-2 minutes it's soft. Add the ground turkey, garlic, salt, Italian seasoning and pepper and cook until ground turkey is browned.

3. Add the canned pumpkin, nutmeg, cinnamon and tomato paste, stir well then. Mix once again, reduce to low heat, cover and let simmer on low.

4. Combine the Parmesan cheese, ricotta cheese, pepper, Italian seasoning and salt in a bowl. Mix until well mixed.

5. Assemble the ravioli by laying out 2 slices of zucchini to form a plus sign. Add the ricotta/Parmesan mixture generously over the middle of the zucchini slices; fold the zucchini, starting from bottom, then the top. Place in an 8 x 8 casserole dish lying upside down. Repeat with the remaining. Top with pumpkin mixture.

9. Bake at 350 degrees F for 30 minutes in the oven. Top with more cheese, if needed.

Nutrition per servings:
Calories: 342kcal; Carbohydrates: 17g; Protein: 29g; Fat: 15g

Mixed Tofu Mushrooms Quiche

Prep time: 20 minutes
Cook time: 60 minutes
Servings: 12

INGREDIENTS

2 tbsp of pickled plum paste or white miso
4 tbsp of sesame tahini
3 lbs of tofu
2 tbsp of tamari
1 lb of chopped broccoli
1 cup of uncooked bulgur wheat
2 yellow onion, chopped
2 tbsp of sesame oil
Pinch of salt
1/2 lb of chopped mushrooms

INSTRUCTIONS

1. Preheat the oven to 350 F. Grease two 9-inch pie pans with non stick spray.
2. Add bulgur and a pinch of salt to two cups of boiling water in a small pot, return to a boil. Reduce heat and cook covered for 15 minutes.
3. Once bulgur timing is complete, remove and add hot bulgur to the prepared pan, slightly press down and baked at 350 F for 12 minutes, or until kind of dry and a bit crusty. Set aside.
4. Heat the oil over medium high heat in a large skillet. Add the onions, mushrooms and broccoli to the pan and cook briefly. Cover with a lid and remove from heat; set aside.

Prepare The Tofu Mixture

5. In a food processor, blend together the tofu, umeboshi paste, tamari and sesame tahini until smooth.
6. Combine the cooked vegetables and tofu mixture in a bowl. Gently toss to combine.
7. Add the vegetable tofu mixture onto the bulgur crust. Place pie pan in the oven and bake for 30 minutes. Remove and set aside for 10 minutes.

Slice into 6 and serve.

Nutrition per servings:
Calories: 190kcal; Carbohydrates: 14g; Protein: 13g; Fat: 8g

Prep time: 15 minutes

Cook time: 15 minutes

Servings: 12 (2 per servings)

INGREDIENTS

1.5 (8 in each tube) tubes of refrigerated crescent rolls, reduced fat

1/2 cup of shredded 2% low fat cheese

1/2 lb of ground turkey (breast meat only)

0.5 envelope of dry onion soup

INSTRUCTIONS

1. Prepare the oven and heat-up to 350 F.

2. Mix the ground turkey meat and dry onion soup together in skillet and brown.

Add in the cheese and mix well until finely blended.

3. Unroll and separate each crescent rolls, cut each triangle into half.

4. Spoon 1 tablespoon of meat mixture in middle of each of the triangle. Fold and seal the edges.

5. Place triangle on a cookie sheet and bake for 15 minutes

Nutrition per servings:

Calories: 155kcal; Carbohydrates: 13g; Protein: 9g; Fat: 7g

Fruit Jelly Tacos

Prep time: 10 minutes

Servings: 2

INGREDIENTS

6 tbsp of regular ricotta cheese

2/3 cup of fresh strawberries, sliced

2 tbsp of low-sugar strawberry jelly

2 small whole wheat tortillas

INSTRUCTIONS

1. Spread the strawberry jelly and ricotta cheese over the tortilla. Add strawberries sliced on top. Roll up the tortilla and serve.

Nutrition per servings:

Calories: 233kcal; Carbohydrates: 22g; Protein: 8g; Fat: 9g

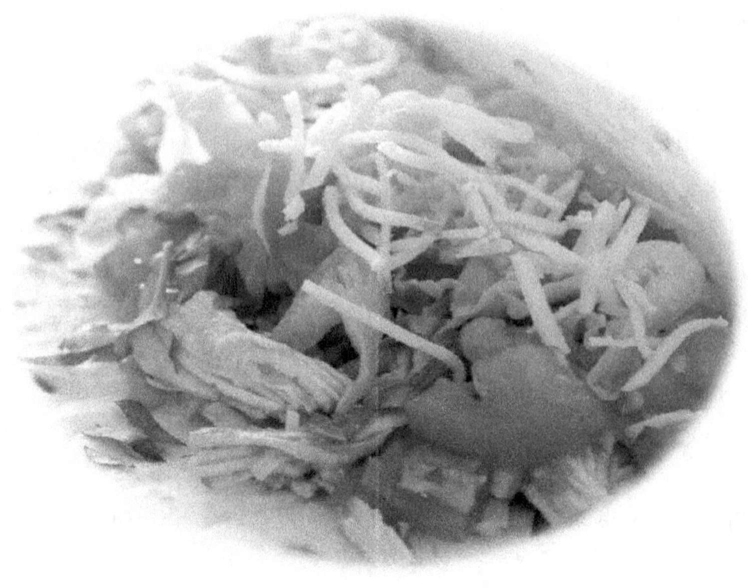

Prep time: 15 minutes

Cook time: 40 minutes

Servings: 3

INGREDIENTS

1/2 tbsp of low-sodium soy sauce

1.5 cups of cooked brown rice

1/2 small onion, sliced (as tolerated)

1 medium green peppers, sliced

1/8 cup of Splenda brown sugar blend

1/6 cup of wine vinegar

1/4 tsp of table salt

1 tbsp of corn starch

Half of 15 oz can of unsweetened pineapple chunks

1/2 lb of lean pork tenderloin, cut thinly into strips

Cooking spray

1/4 cup of water

INSTRUCTIONS

1. Cook the pork tenderloin in a frying pan sprayed with non stick cooking spray over medium heat until its golden brown. Remove pork and drain fat from cooking, set pork aside.

2. Drain the juice from the pineapple chunks and set aside.

3. In a small bowl, mix the water, soy sauce, reserved pineapple juice, cornstarch, vinegar, sugar and salt. Add mixture into the pan and cook for about 2 minutes until sauce is thickened.

4. Add in the pork and cook further over low heat, stirring occasionally for about 30 minutes until meat is tender.

5. Add in the pineapple chunks, peppers and onion and cook for another 5 minutes. Serve over rice.

Nutrition per servings:

Calories: 248kcal; Carbohydrates: 28g; Protein: 18g; Fat: 3.5g

Mixed Veggies Pork Stew

Prep time: 30 minutes

Cook time: 8 hours

Servings: 2-3

INGREDIENTS

1/2 tsp of pepper

1/2 cup of water

1 cup of desired assorted vegetables

5 ounces diced tomatoes drained of excess liquid

Half of 1 can of chipotle peppers in adobo sauce

1/8 cup of part-skim ricotta cheese

0.5 pound of country ribs

1 bay leave

1/2 tsp of ground cumin

1/2 tsp of salt

1/2 tsp of ground coriander

INSTRUCTIONS

1. Add 1/2 cup of water, coriander, country ribs, pepper, cumin, salt and bay leaves into your slow cooker. Cook for about 6 hours on low.

2. Remove the meat form the cooker, remove bones from meat and shred with two forks. Discard the bay leaves.

3. Combine the diced tomatoes and about 2 chipotle peppers (depending on how spicy you like it) in a blender and blend. Transfer to the cooker along with the assorted vegetables. Cook further for 2 hours.

4. Serve a bowl, topped with ricotta cheese and garnish with a little cilantro.

Ready time: 5 minutes

Servings: 4

INGREDIENTS

(Optional) pinch of Salt

2 (15 oz each) can of canned pinto or kidney beans

Green or Red Tabasco sauce, to taste

2 lime Juice

INSTRUCTIONS

1. Mix together the entire ingredients food processor or blend with hand mixer until smooth.

Nutrition per servings:

Calories: 198kcal; Carbohydrates: Protein: 11.5g; Fat: 1.5g

Crumble Apple Almonds Ramekins

Prep time: 10 minutes

Cook time: 15 minutes

Servings: 4

INGREDIENTS

2 tbsp of no-calorie sweetener

6 tbsp of no-calorie sweetener

4 small Granny Smith apples (peeled, cored and sliced)

1/2 tsp of apple pie spice

2 tbsp of butter

2 tbsp of sliced almonds

1 cup of high fiber cereal

INSTRUCTIONS

1. Prepare the oven and heat-up to 350 F.

2. Coat a non-stick frying pan with cooking spray. Heat over a medium high heat until it's hot. Add in the apples slices, pie spice and sweetener

and cook for about 3 minutes until apples are tender. Place the mixture into ramekins.

3. Pulse the almonds, cereal, butter and sweetener in a mini-food processor until well combined. Scoop mixture into each ramekin.

4. Bake in the oven for 35 minutes at 350 degrees or until filling bubbles on top and top is crispy.

Tuna Patties With Lemon Greek yogurt

Prep time: 5 minutes

Cook time: 10 minutes

Servings: 4

INGREDIENTS

Pepper, dill and dried mustard, to taste

1/2 tbsp of minced onion

1/8 cup of chopped water chestnuts, diced red pepper or capers

1/8 cup of grated carrot

8 Wheat thins crackers, crushed

2 egg whites

2 (3-oz) canned of tuna in water

INSTRUCTIONS

1. Combine the entire ingredients in a mixing bowl.

2. Use your hands to form mixture into 8 patties.

3. Coat a medium sized pan with nonstick spray and heat over a medium high heat.

4. Place the patties and cook for 2-3 minutes per side until golden brown on both sides. Serve with a dollop of fat-free Greek yogurt and lemon squeeze.

Nutrition per servings:
Calories: 80kcal; Carbohydrates: 4g; Protein: 12g; Fat: 1g

Peanut Spinach Garbanzo Stew

Prep time: 15 minutes
Cook time: 40 minutes
Servings: 8

INGREDIENTS

2 cups of creamy peanut butter
6 cans of garbanzo beans (15 oz. cans)
1/4-1/2 cup of sriracha sauce
8 oz of tomato paste
4 cups of water
8 cups of baby spinach
2 tsp of garam masala
1 tsp of tumeric
1 tsp of ground cumin
2 tbsp of olive oil
4 minced garlic clove
6 diced tomatoes
2 small diced yellow onions
1 tsp of ground coriander
Salt and pepper to taste
2 cans of peas and carrots (25 oz total)

INSTRUCTIONS

1. Heat olive oil over medium heat in a soup pot placed over medium heat. Add the onions, garlic and tomatoes and sauté 2-3 minutes.

2. Add in the carrots, peas, water with the spices, stir well; reduce to low heat. Cover with the lid and bring to a boil.

3. Blend the tomato paste and peanut butter in a mixing bowl until well blended. Use a little of the veggie mixture to thin out the peanut mixture, and then add into the soup pot. Stir well then add the hot sauce, starting with about 2 tbsp.

4. Add in the baby spinach and garbanzo beans and stir.

Nutrition per servings:
Calories: 266kcal; Carbohydrates: 18g; Protein: 31g; Fat: 12g

Prep time: 5 minutes

Cook time: 5 minutes

Servings: 8

INGREDIENTS

2 tbsp of olive oil

8 (4 ounces each) orange roughy fillets

1/2 tsp of ground pepper

16 medium lemon wedges

2 tbsp of Dijon mustard

6 tbsp of lemon juice

INSTRUCTIONS

1. Clean your baking sheet or broiler rack and line with foil, then spray with non-stick cooking spray.

2. Combine together the olive oil, mustard, lemon juice and ground pepper in a bowl and stir well. Transfer the fish over to the prepared baking sheet or broiler rack. Brush 1/2 of the mixture over fish fillets. Broil fish until it starts to flakes easily, about 5 minutes.

3. Drizzle the remaining 1/2 mixture and pepper over to taste. Garnish with lemon wedges.

Nutrition per servings:

Calories: 114kcal; Carbohydrates: 2.5g; Protein: 17g; Fat: 4g

Brown Rice Chicken Bean Casserole

Prep time: 15 minutes

Cook time: 1 hour 25 minutes

Servings: 4

INGREDIENTS

7.5 oz can of black beans, drained

1/6 cup of shredded carrots

2 oz can of diced green chilies

1/2 medium thinly sliced zucchini

1 cups of low fat Swiss cheese, shredded

1/8 tsp of cayenne pepper

1/6 cup of brown rice

8 ounces of cooked skinless, boneless chicken breast, chopped into small pieces

1/6 cup of diced onion

1/4 cup of sliced mushrooms

1/2 tbsp of olive oil

1/2 cup of vegetable broth

1/4 tsp of cumin

INSTRUCTIONS

1. Cook the broth and rice into a pot over medium high heat, once it comes to a boil, turn heat down, cover and let it simmer for 45 minutes or until rice is cooked and soft. Set aside.

2. Prepare your oven and heat to 350 F.

3. Heat the olive oil over medium heat in skillet, add the onions and cook until tender. Add in chicken, mushrooms, zucchini and seasonings, stir everything together. Cook stirring until chicken is heated and zucchini is lightly browned.

4. Combine the chicken, rice, zucchini, onion, beans, mushrooms, carrots, and 1/2 cup of Swiss cheese and chilies in large bowl.

5. Add the mixture into a large lightly greased casserole dish, sprinkle with remaining cheese.

6. Cover loosely in foil and bake in preheated oven for 30 minutes. Uncover, bake further for 10 minutes or until browned lightly.

Nutrition per servings:
Calories: 267kcal; Carbohydrates: 16g; Protein: 31g; Fat: 6g

Meaty Cabbage Rolls

Prep time: 15 minutes
Cook time: 1 hour 10 minutes
Servings: 3
INGREDIENTS
1 tsp of Italian or Oregano seasoning
1/4 medium diced onion (if you can tolerate)
1 tsp of garlic powder
1/2 lbs of 93% lean ground turkey
1 cups of tomato sauce
1/2 head of cabbage, remove individual leaves
1 medium diced carrot
1/2 tsp of olive oil
1/6 cup of instant brown Rice Minute, or any whole grain rice
INSTRUCTIONS
1. Prepare the oven and heat to 350°F.
2. Wash the cabbage clean and blanch in boiling water for 30 seconds.
3. Prepare rice as instructed in package directed.
4. Meanwhile, heat olive oil in a large skillet over medium heat. Add the carrots and onions, cook stirring until fragrance and slightly soft. Add in the turkey and cook it's until browned. Add the garlic powders and Italian or Oregano seasonings.
5. Add the cooked rice with the meat mixture into the pan. Add half cup of rice meat mixture into middle of one cabbage leaf. Roll up and seal both ends. Repeat with the remaining.

6. Place the seam side down of cabbage rolls into your baking dish, resting on one another so they won't unroll.

7. Spread the tomato sauce over top of the cabbage rolls, spilling over to the bottom of baking dish.

8. Place baking dish in the oven and bake for about 35-45 minutes. Let cool for 10 minutes before you serve.

Nutrition per servings:
Calories: 174kcal; Carbohydrate

Moist Boneless Chicken

Prep time: 10 minutes
Cook time: 40 minutes
Servings: 6

INGREDIENTS

1/8 of any light mayo of choice
3/4 cups of whole wheat Italian bread crumbs
1.5 lbs of boneless, skinless chicken breasts

INSTRUCTIONS

1. Prepare the oven and heat-up to 425 F. Line your baking sheet with foil.

2. Brush the chicken with the light mayonnaise thoroughly.

3. Coat the chicken in a bowl of bread crumbs until chicken coated.

4. Bake the chicken in the oven for 40-45 minutes or until cooked through.

Nutrition per servings:
Calories: 233kcal; Carbohydrates: 6g; Protein: 37g; Fat: 5g